Poppy Seed

Revealing the Roots of the Opioid Epidemic

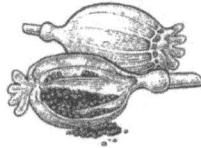

Other books by Anthony Anonimo:

Lord of the Wind

Dark Corner of the Mind

Poppy Seed

Revealing the Roots of the Opioid Epidemic

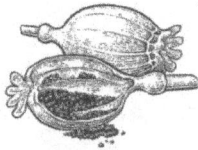

Anthony Anonimo

HenschelHAUS Publishing, Inc.
Milwaukee, Wisconsin

Published by

HenschelHAUS Publishing, Inc.

www.henschelhausbooks.com

ISBN: 978159598-549 –1

E-ISBN: 978159598-550-7

Library of Congress Number: 2017944383

Printed in the United States.

This book is dedicated to:

Benny Sicilia, lost to OxyContin
Bobby Peret, lost to heroin
Jacob De Voe, lost to heroin

And all those unfortunate souls who lost
their lives through the deception
of addiction

Papaver Somniferum

If we look back in the history of life and the events that alter our world seemingly forever, it is interesting that the beginnings of change happen in a split second. And it is that very split second that mushrooms into the making of eternal changes in our society.

And so it is that man virtually took what seemed to be something as tiny as a "Poppy Seed" and turned it into a bed of horror, a horror that will live on forever in eternity.

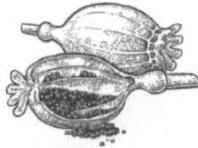

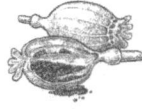

CHAPTER ONE

There was a time in my early teens that I tried smoking this stuff a friend of mine had, called Afghanistan opiated hashish. I had been smoking pot and hash for probably a year or so previously, but never experienced anything like the opiated hash. I remember thinking that we had discovered a secret treasure unknown to most people. That stuff was like a gentle orgasm which lasted for hours. It seemed that everything else in life back then, would just have to take a back seat to this stuff. From then on it seemed I was on a mission.

Well, unknown to me that stuff was no secret to the rest of the world. As I began to read up on opium in some library books, I found some very interesting facts about it. And here I thought I had made some secret discovery.

Apparently opium was so popular there were wars started over the stuff back in the mid 1800's. In fact, Fossil remains of poppy-seed cake and poppy-pods had been found in Neolithic Swiss lake-dwellings dating from over 4,000 years ago. Poppy images appear in Egyptian pictography and Roman sculptures.

In my research I found that the First Opium War was launched by the biggest, richest, and perhaps most aggressive drug cartel the world has ever known, which the "British Empire" was. The Chinese were defeated. They were forced to sign the Treaty of Nanjing in 1842. The British required that the opium trade be allowed to continue; that the Chinese pay a large settlement and open five new ports to foreign trade; and that China cede Hong Kong to Britain. I guess oil isn't the only thing that started wars.

History says that famous guys like Wild Bill Hickok and Kit Carson actually frequented opium dens more often than saloons. The stereo-typed picture we have of the cowhand belly up to the bar drinking whiskey straight after a long hard ride on the dusty trail is only part of the story of the old west. Oftentimes the cowhand was not bellying up to a bar at all. He was in a prone position in a dimly lit room smoking opium in the company of an oriental prostitute. It wasn't uncommon for some of these cowboys to spend several days and nights at a time in these dens in a constant dream-state, eventually becoming physically addicted to the drug.

According to history the real knock down shootouts back in the old west were the results of alcohol, not drugs. Alcohol was one of the major sources of violence and death during this period. Eventually, however, opium was promoted as a cure for alcoholism by the late 1800's.

Back then physicians commonly believed that the poppy plant was of divine origin; opium was interesting enough called the Sacred Anchor of Life, Milk of Paradise, and Destroyer of Grief.

Thomas Sydenham, the 17th-century pioneer of English medicine, wrote....

"Among the remedies which it has pleased Almighty God to give to man to relieve his sufferings, none is so universal and as efficacious as opium."

Indeed opium was probably the world's first authentic antidepressant. If you look at all of the phrases used for opium dating as far back as 4,000 years ago, it's called "the stone of immortality"

Some other terms used to describe opium were, "the Hand of God" "God's Own Paradise" "the plant of joy."

My experience with opium and its derivatives say it's the devils brew disguised as the God of pleasure. Look, if the ancient Egyptians and Romans took the time to etch the poppy's image in stone, you know it was important.

The late Lenny Bruce said..."I may die young, but it's like kissing God"

Even Thomas Jefferson was known to have cultivated opium poppies at his garden in Monticello.

I guess it was in the mid 1800's that some magic man who they called a pharmacist began to mix stuff up using opium in his quest to make some voodoo medicine. He was apparently creating colorful dyes from coal tar. The company expanded its operations with coal-tar being the main product. With price conventions and the availability of raw materials diminishing, the company invested in diversifying its production range.

In 1888, a new substance synthesized by the company's chemists became the company's first commercial medicine. Apparently they had been using crude natural materials like opium, the dried milky juice of poppy seed pods. Well, this young German pharmacist named Friedrich had first applied chemical analysis to plant drugs, by purifying in 1805 the main active ingredient of opium. Apparently after testing the stuff out and falling in love with it, he likened it to Morpheus, the Greek god of dreams. He gave his drug the name 'morphium' which later became morphine.

Perhaps appropriately, the discoverer of morphine was in due course nominated for academic honors, and rightfully so. Hell, I give him a Tony award!

There was another family business headed by a guy named George, who turned his pharmacy business into a big supplier of some of these new products, derived from opium. The one in particular, being morphine, was being widely used in the American Civil War and also in the Franco - Prussian war. Got pain...no problem...morphine was now available. And in combination with the invention of the hypodermic syringe, there's no waiting in aisle one.

In the late 1890's a German company had some very talented pharmacologists that began to purify plant derived drugs. They began to modify these drugs by adding acetyl groups to make them more effective. The two most famous drugs known today, heroin and aspirin, came out of this company.

Heroin, the first semi-synthetic opiate, was originally synthesized in 1874, but was apparently shelved until its rediscovery in 1897 by Felix Hoffmann at the Bayer pharmaceutical company in Elberfeld, Germany. Heroin was initially marketed as a non-addictive morphine substitute and cough medicine for children. By 1902, 5% of the company's profits, and "heroin" had attracted much attention.

Ironically enough, heroin derived its name from the word 'heroic'. It was presented to the world by introducing it as a cough, chest, and lung medicine. Painful diseases such as pneumonia and tuberculosis were the leading causes of death at that time, so when all else failed heroin was used to alleviate suffering. Hell, I would have said I was suffering.

In 1898 a German chemical company began bottling this drug (heroin) and it was flooding its way into Britain.

In fact, it was right before the turn of the century that heroin had replaced morphine as the drug of choice used by most physicians. Early in its implementation it was prescribed for relieving coughs and producing sleep. Heroin was tested on phthisic patients, where it was initially given orally in doses of 5 and 10 mg. And the doctor who originally oversaw the testing noted no unpleasant reactions; and of course the patients liked it. In fact they reportedly continued to take it even after this doc ceased to prescribe it. Now why the hell couldn't I have lived back then?

Heroin mimics the action of natural chemicals, endorphins, produced by the body in response to pain. Endorphins are small-chain peptides that activate our endogenous opioid receptors. Opioid receptors are proteins embedded in the cell membrane; opioid agonists bind to the receptors to initiate their effects. The highest density of opioid receptors is found in the limbic system. Their activation produces feelings of happiness, relaxation, fearlessness and tolerance to pain. Endorphins are hundreds or even thousands of times more potent than morphine on a molar basis.

The consumption of heroin is marked by a euphoric rush, a warm feeling of relaxation, a sense of security and protection, and a dissipation of pain, fear, hunger, tension and anxiety. When heroin is snorted or smoked, the rush is intense and orgasmic. Subjectively, time may slow down. Any sense of anger, frustration or aggression disappears. Users enjoy the feeling of "being wrapped in God's warmest blanket".

In 1899 a physician by the name of Horatio reported that heroin dosages had to be increased with usage to remain effective. It was during this period that the preoccupation with morphine addiction, prompted some doctors to advocate treatment by heroin in 'demorphinisation'. It wasn't until this practice was criticized by J. Jarrige in 1902, who began to observe that heroin withdrawal symptoms were even worse than those of morphine.

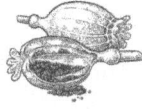

CHAPTER TWO

Well, here the hell we sit some hundred plus years later; with a similar problem with OxyContin, Fentanyl, and methadone. Does anyone really want this stuff gone and done with? Or, is there just too much money in this trade? My answer...ABSOLUTELY YES!

It was in 1903 the stuff (heroin) was exposed for what the hell it was. The Alabama Medical Journal had published an article entitled 'The Heroin Habit another Curse', and even after that, some physicians were still reluctant to abandon this highly effective drug. In 1911, some Doctor wrote in the Kentucky Medical Journal: 'I feel that bringing charges against heroin is almost like questioning the fidelity of a good friend. I have used it with good results.'

And I would contend that it became his best friend. Maybe his only friend eventually.

As for me it didn't take long at all; My Heroin and I were like two pees in a pod; I never really did want to break off our relationship. It was like a wild fling that I just couldn't stop seeking day after day regardless of promises to quit moments earlier.

The United States was the first country that heroin addiction had become an epidemic. By the late nineteenth century other countries experienced the same serious problems. Germany and Britain quickly enacted laws to control narcotics, but in the US it was left up to each individual state to make medical regulations, as to have it available only by prescription. So heroin, morphine, and cocaine, were still readily available over the counter in a bordering state without regulation.

By the year 1900 the United States was believed to have at least a quarter million addicts, or "junkies" (the term "junkie" originated from heroin addicts stealing redeemable metals to supply their habits)

Hell, in 1906 the United States government had to pass regulation that made companies label the contents of their products. There were companies putting heroin, cocaine, and opium in many over the counter 'cures', even for babies. And when you looked at the labels of these remedies there was no mention of the secret ingredients, and in many cases they denied it.

I can tell you by way of first-hand knowledge that opium was, and still is used in remedies for curing diarrhea. That too I can tell you works wonders. I remember times back when I was using heavily that I would go almost 2 weeks without taking a dump. You could say I was really full of shit back then.

It also seemed that without the use of the Internet and cell phones information flowed much slower back then. It was pretty common that the majority of the public was unaware that opium derived ingredients were inside quite a few items behind the counter pharmacies and in some cases over the counter medications.

It's believed that by the year 1910 there were nearly 200,000 heroin addicts in New York City alone. And with drug usage hitting epidemic proportions throughout the country the United States government passed a law called the "Harrison Narcotics Act". Under this law, it became illegal to own, use, or be addicted to illicitly-obtained narcotics. Doctors and pharmacists were required to register and pay a tax on all prescriptions. This was the beginning of arrests for drug abuse. In some areas, the majority of prisoners in federal facilities would be incarcerated there on drug charges.

What is amazing looking back, is that heroin had become so appealing that opium trade controls were actually added to the Treaty of Versailles. That goes to show just how powerful this stuff really was that it would become a major item added to a world renowned peace treaty. Heroin had become enormously popular just that fast, probably second to gold. And I guess you could say that it was like gold to the soul. Heroin just seemed to have an instant fix for pain, both physically and psychologically. No one on earth ever experienced such a phenomenon.

In 1924, the deputy commissioner of the New York Police reported that 94% of all crimes were being committed by heroin addicts. Soon after, the drug was outlawed for both medical and illicit use. The League of Nations followed with more restrictions, and the manufacturing and export of heroin began to be controlled.

The regulations and bans that were put into place just moved heroin production from factories in Europe to clandestine labs in China. Then drug channels to Europe and the United States began to be controlled by organized crime in Europe, better known as the "French Connection" which importing of unrefined heroin to France, where it went to refinement plants before being shipped to Eastern US cities and throughout Europe.

Heroin supplies into the US were restricted due to increased security when WW II began. Most heroin addicts in the US were no longer able to get the drug and the number of addicts dropped. But the new pattern only lasted until the end of World War II. Then the mafia and other black market syndicates went back into business. And shortly after that, when the United States government intervened in conflicts in Southeast Asia, it put millions of soldiers right smack in the middle of heroin manufacturers and traffickers.

Heroin manufacturers moved from Turkey to Southeast Asia due to complicated political plays around the time that the CIA (Central Intelligence Agency) was created. It could have been coincidence that US government officials began infiltration throughout the world, but it is ironic to say the least. That all occurred in the wake of World War II. It was then, American and European crime syndicates transferred their supplier routes to Southeast Asia where everything seemed to converge, thus creating the "Golden Triangle"

Over the next twenty years, about four million American military men and women would be stationed in the area of the "Golden Triangle" or nearby. It is believed to be one of the major influences that would eventually lead to America's heroin addiction rates skyrocketing to numbers that had never been seen before.

Even with regulations, laws, criminalization, preventive education, you name it, this stuff continued to wreak havoc throughout the world.

* * * * *

In 1937 German scientists came up with a synthetic opiate 'cure' so to speak, named Dolphine, or Methadone, is what we also know it as.

According to popular legend, its substitute, methadone, was initially christened Dolophine in honor of Adolf Hitler. In reality, the name comes from the Latin dolor, meaning "pain", and fin, meaning "end": hence "end of pain".

Germany began selling it to the US in mass quantities. This nasty drug is believed to be more addictive than heroin. And I for one can attest to that. It is some wicked shit. So, in the quest for a cure, things get worse instead of better, not to mention just a bigger variety to choose from.

Hell, one fact is that Methadone has proven to create jobs opening clinics throughout the United States. And I can tell you first hand, they are keeping their jobs. What junkie is going to stop going to a clinic that is giving out free 'Synthetic Heroin'?

As I have mentioned so many times before, 'where the hell is our drug czar'? Heroin use is again on the rise. But, it seems to be another big business with a very lucrative profit margin. And why again is the United States military guarding the Poppy fields in Afghanistan? Shit, over 85 percent of the worlds heroin production is coming out of that place.

The US investigation of a Mexican cartel in Guerrero, Mexico shows an alarming fact. From 2009 to 2015 the influx of heroin has nearly doubled. The place of origin, Mexico, with the heroin supply coming into the US has grown from about 39 percent to over fifty percent in just three years.

Mexican farmers in Guererro went from growing Avocados, to growing Poppies, and by 2015 heroin has become the major export, with nearly 90 percent of the product going to the US. And most of the heroin being brought into the US by way of the cartel runners who distribute most all of the heroin to small rural areas of the US. Using the smaller rural areas as distribution points has been quite lucrative for the cartels, as well as being much safer to distribute without stepping on other crime syndicates in places like Chicago and New York, though it does eventually find its way there too.

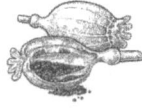

CHAPTER THREE

Heroin use in the US has nearly doubled since 2009, according to sources within our drug enforcement agencies. In 2014, the United Nations reported that 1 in 25 people under the age of 15 have tried heroin. This is an alarming figure when you think about it.

Southeast Asia's heroin production has tripled since 2006. That's only eight years that the distribution of this stuff has tripled. And, the heroin coming out of the "Golden Triangle " mainly by Laos farmers, is reportedly more pure than the stuff coming out of Afghanistan.

And though the vast majority of heroin that floods our earth still hails from Afghanistan, nearly 85 percent, it is believed that between the "Golden Triangle", Mexico, and Latin America, the harvesting and processing of poppies have nearly tripled in just the past decade.

Now, much of the many government surveillance efforts have certainly helped in identifying where the poppy fields are located, by way of aerial observation where these poppy farms are located. However, what's happening with the cartels that run these farms and process heroin when raided, seized, and destroyed, the cartel moves the farm laborers to set up Meth labs. The Meth labs are nearly impossible to locate until it's too late. By the time foot patrols of the government run agencies in these areas locate them, they're way too far behind the proverbial eight ball to make even a dent in production and distribution. It's kind of like a bacteria that once it is eradicated, it seems to get smarter, and grow a new armor of sorts, protecting itself from elimination. The people running these operations are no fools, in fact, they may just be shrewder than some of the top business executives on earth. Their corporations too are publicly traded, so to speak, however in a much different way. They ain't no fools.

It's very interesting to say the least that whenever there is military intervention in Afghanistan, heroin supplies, use, and deaths, reach alarming highs. Now whether it's corrupt politicians, military brass, or the CIA, I always say "here we go again".

I remember back in the 1970's when The Soviet Union invaded Afghanistan. That's when I first saw the trends. You could bet that some US crime syndicates were in high level dealings with the Russian mafia, or government, if you will. In those days heroin use spiked considerably.

Now, when you look at the heroin production coming from Afghanistan, where nearly 85% of the worlds heroin supply originates, it again is a glaring phenomenon.

In 2001 the heroin production out of Afghanistan was at an all-time low. Then, ironically 9-11 came about. Well, the US military just happened to see to it that they invade Afghanistan to look for Osama. It was kind of like finding Waldo. I sometimes wonder if the guy even existed.

Well, sure enough one year after the military intervention into the region, mainly Afghanistan, our soldiers needed to guard the poppy fields. If we're not guarding oil, we're tending to opium fields.

What happened in 2002? You probably guessed it, the heroin production out of Afghanistan spiked right back up. In fact, it jumped nearly 70% in one short year, and has grown considerably since then year after year.

It's all about one guy? Bull shit, I say. Are we that naïve that one freakin guy lured us into a total invasion of that entire region of the world.

Well, if it's one guy we're looking for, it's much easier to say "Damn, we just missed him" ok. Then we keep looking for this cave dweller. Ok, now we got him, but now we need to be sure his cousins and friends don't give us a hard time. All the while our military is guarding the opium fields. You never know, his family and friends might be hiding there. What a freaking joke.

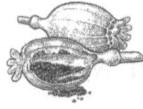

CHAPTER FOUR

Someone once asked me what I thought it was that draws so many people to heroin in the first place. My response was then and is now that there are a vast number of reasons. When I look back on my history with heroin I can see that it was a combination of so many things which all added up to the same end, dissatisfaction with life itself. What I will tell you is this…it's anything from broken dreams to massive success that strikes the majority of people, some time in their lives. For me, I'd say broken dreams, insecurity, and worthlessness. I can't answer for everyone, but what I can tell you is this, if you add all of the reasons given for using heroin, from all of the people that have ever used it throughout history, it always seems to come to the same conclusion, discontentment.

There are some of us that have had a distain for life from the beginning, because of a troubled childhood of some sort.

When people choose their poison whether it is alcohol, marijuana, cocaine, barbiturates, or even sniffing glue, the overwhelming reason always seems to point to an unsettled life. Whether it's the stress of everyday life at work, an unsatisfactory relationship, and poverty, loss of loved ones, or just plain boredom, the real pitfall is that if it's heroin or other opiates that you choose as your savior, you lose, hands down. The reason you lose is that it makes you feel so damn good, there's nothing in the mood altering world that can pale in comparison.

How many times could someone say that they've indulged in something that made them puke their guts out seconds after doing it, and never find it disgusting while in the moment? With alcohol, when most people begin to heave it almost always comes with an "oh my god, help me please stop!" But with heroin, it's much the opposite because absolute euphoria sets in. You never felt so good. And not only is it physically addicting, it's extremely psychologically and even emotionally addicting.

Now, when I put this analogy out there I can only imagine that it may sound as though I am enticing people in anguish, drawing people with a loss of direction in life, or even someone with plain curiosity, but the fact remains that this shit will change your life forever. And the outcome is never, ever, good. It is in fact a dead end in so many different ways. Relationships are crushed, families are torn apart, financial stability is ripped away, and the user's mental health and personality are forever ridden with guilt, if they survive that is.

My analogy is this:

The heroin addict is like a tornado roaring his way through the lives of others.

Hearts are broken and sweet relationships die if ever they existed. Affections will have been uprooted. Selfish and inconsiderate habits will have kept everyone affected by the addict in turmoil. And if the addict is so fortunate as to live through the dark turmoil, which is likened to being in the eye of a hurricane, it is then and only then, can they make the necessary amends to themselves and the ones they've harmed. That is in fact if there is any chance of redemption from the toll it most likely took on the innocent bystanders in their lives.

An addict will lie, steal, cheat, and repeat. And if you think by holding an addicts hand until the physical withdrawal has lifted is the end, think again. It is only the beginning. The road to recovery after true heroin addiction is a never ending task. It takes tenacity, hard work, and consistency. And as far as consistency goes in a junkies life? I truly believe that the only consistency an addict adheres to is the fact that they make sure they get their fix. And it is regardless of any possible obstacle in the way of getting it.

I don't care if it's a person, place, or thing, in the way of that fix, it will be run over like it were hit by a late freight train. All the apologies might come afterwards, but like I said, after. During the moments of active addiction you, the innocent bystander, are nothing more than an obstacle, believe me.

And for the apologies, forget about it. All the "I'm so sorry(s) I stole your money" "I'm Sorry I hurt you" I say "F*** you junkie, No you're not." A junkie doesn't care about a damn thing, except for the fact that they didn't get more from their victims. It's just a sore fact of active addiction.

It is almost as if that once that poppy seed infiltrates the junkie's brain, the only hope of keeping it at bay is by not feeding it.

It's like that of another story I once heard sitting around a table of recovering drug addicts and alcoholics one day, in Lower Manhattan. It is actually an old Cherokee legend.

It is of an old grandfather Cherokee teaching his grandson about life. He said to his grandson, "There is a fight going on in my head".

"There is a terrible fight between two wolves. One is evil, full of anger, resentment, envy, sorrow, regret, arrogance, self-pity, ego, guilt, false pride, and lies.

The other wolf is good, he is joy, peace, love, hope, serenity, humility, kindness, benevolence, empathy, generosity, truth, compassion, and faith."

"The same fight is going on inside of you, and inside the head of everyone else on earth", said the grandfather.

The grandson thought about it for a moment, and asked, "Which wolf will win?" And the grandfather responded, "The one you feed."

I'd never heard that story before that day, but it stuck in my head ever since. And when I think about it, I find it very interesting. It dawned on me that it's been so very easy for me to feed the evil wolf because of the fact that it has such a louder growl and harder bite. It's almost like the saying of the squeaky wheel gets the grease. It's so easy for me to appease the louder of the two, even though the other can be so peaceful and serene.

I guess what it tells me is something that has been mentioned from the beginning of mankind. It's that negative thoughts carry more weight. And what's so intriguing about it is, that I would think that paying attention to the negative thoughts would lighten their proverbial weight. But I guess that paying credence to the negative thoughts is actually feeding the thing that I am attempting to rid myself of. And, I guess it also makes sense to why it's so hard to give attention to good and peaceful thoughts and feelings. They're already good, so it takes a whole different approach when I contemplated how to feed them. I guess the proper way is to actually feed off the good and starve the negative, best I can.

It's that moment of truth that lies beyond the elimination of the physical withdrawals and acceptance of the reality in knowing you're sick and tired of being sick and tired, that you've truly begun on the path to sobriety. Not to mention an addict is probably going to be nursing the physical damage the body went through during that God awful war. It is then and only then that true recovery can begin. If and when a recovering addict has reached that point of truth, they will undoubtedly recognize the damage they actually did to themselves and others. There are destructive behavioral patterns that had slowly developed during the days of utter deception which need correction. Along with so many bad habits that go with that corrupt lifestyle.

The aftermath goes something like this, a story I once read, and it says:

I feel a man is unthinking when he says that sobriety is enough.

He is like the farmer who came up out of his tornado shelter to find his home ruined.

To his wife, he remarks,

"Don't see anything the matter here, Ma. Ain't it grand the wind stopped blowing?"

Well, truth be told, cleaning up is only the first step. Now I won't deny that it is definitely the only step to say a person is clean. But...sober? Absolutely not! Anyone who tells you that, is either lying to themselves or just plain misinformed. Then again, there are those unfortunates that just cannot, or will not, grasp the fact that their addiction didn't happen overnight.

It takes rigorous honesty of looking inside oneself to correct the stinking thinking, the terrible habits, and the tainted relationships, to the admission of powerlessness over people, places, and things. It's the admission that the needed change is within oneself and nothing more.

So, if you're looking for a deterrent to eliminate someone from even entertaining the thought of trying it, that too is simple in theory. For guidelines in raising our youth, it's this, keep them talking and keep them busy. Do your best in helping them pinpoint a purpose for their lives? Without purpose, they are probably lost and whether it's heroin, alcohol, other drugs, or just plain discontentment which WILL in fact lead to depression and hopelessness.

You may ask me, "If you're so smart and knowledgeable about this subject how'd you become who you are?" The only answer I have is this, I'm still alive, and I have no incentive to relive that life other than my attempt to give back to society what I learned while defying life, tarnishing my loved ones, and living a life of complete insanity. That lifestyle assisted in my feeling of embarrassment and my quest to right the wrong the only way I know how, by passing my message.

You may also ask, what do you know about raising our youth? Well I don't, in fact I have no freaking clue other than a practice I observed in watching successful people, and successful families. And what I've learned has given me hope that our world's future may just have a chance. The unfortunate thing is that I may have found out later than I wish I had. Like my father always said to me... "You'll learn" and holy shit, did I.

In the success I've observed in many of the families seems to be based on many different things. There are things like sports, music, forensics, and the many other positive and habitual activities that many parents instill in their childrearing. Now what I can tell you is this, through the years there have been many people who came from successful families, such as the ones I mentioned. And yes, there are some people from these said families who have become addicts. But what I can also tell you is that from my observation and what statistical data will tell you is that these same people have a better than 50 percent chance to rise up and into recovery.

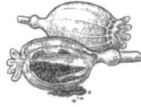

CHAPTER FIVE

My world began in the summer of 1955, in the little city of Milwaukee Wisconsin. I was just another little boy brought into this glorious planet of promise and beauty.

I remember my rides in an old stroller my mother pushed along a pathway along a creek near our home. On our travels I saw the beautiful blue sky up above and a magnificent variety of birds. The birds each sang their own language almost as if they were saying 'is this great, or what'. In the background I could hear the water flowing over the rocks in the nearby brook. And the leaves were all seeming to flutter their own dance to the light wind of the day.

While the sights and sounds of those days made me feel so energetic, yet peaceful, and invigorating though calming. These are feelings and memories that I would never, ever, forget.

The only sad part of those days was the fact these little jaunts into paradise always came to an end.

Looking back now, I realize I may have been, and still am now, a whole hell of a lot different than other people. It seems as though my appreciation for life and its beauty only lasted for the moment I lived it. Contrary to how I see other people's admiration for the allures of life, which seems to live on in satisfaction, I myself felt disappointed.

I wanted more. When I encountered beauty and good feelings I craved that it be endless. I seemed to have a thirst that was never satisfied with just a taste. In thinking back, I believe it may be just unappreciative. It's difficult to appreciate something that didn't fulfill my endless thirst. If something is endless, that's just what the hell it is.

I remember as a kid, one day my older brother told me that God could make anything. Then he said, He can even make a stick with one end. That one made me wonder occasionally, even to this day. A stick with one end? Hmmm. WTF.

Well, with my constant appetite for pleasure and the passion toward always wanting more, I headed out in my pursuit of happiness in this insane world of ours.

The problem with my quest of what I defined as contentment was probably the pursuit of the stick with one end. Only my pleasure seeking began with a dick with one end. And that one end always seemed to create a multitude of troubling aftershocks in my life.

Yes...one was too many because I could never settle for something I liked, without going for two. And a thousand was never enough. Why stop if it feels good.

It was in the summer of 1969 that I discovered a plethora of women, booze, and drugs. I also wanted more, and I wanted them all simultaneously.

It was when I discovered heroin and cocaine that my life took on a whole new meaning. I was hooked. I lied, stole, cheated, and repeated. Needless to say due to my addictive personality I went nonstop from the moment my eyes opened to the world. And I never stopped until I was passed out cold.

At age 16 I continued to do what I thought was expected by society in the way of going to school and working at a minimum as to keep up the image of a 'normal' person. But in reality my mind was truly invested in the dark side of the other life I lived.

We would highjack a few liquor and cigarette trucks, distributed pills and pot, and sold anything obtained illegally with the likes of guns, TV's, and stereos. I felt I had a purpose. Then with all of the guilt I incurred that I could justify drinking and drugging. Is that messed up or what?

By the age of 19, I was in way over my head and began to completely drown myself with cocaine, heroin, and morphine. I had no clue what was up, down, right or wrong. On the surface I continued to comply with society the best I possibly could to keep a righteous face on my life's activities by getting clean for short periods of time. But what I didn't know then was that I was only fooling myself. It was like clockwork that every time I relapsed, this allergy of mine seemed to result in finding myself breaking out in handcuffs.

I very quickly found that heroin had stolen my heart, and it also took my soul with it. I was an absolute mess to put it lightly.

My life into and through my twenties was like a blur. When society says that life in ones twenties is for progress and development of molding a successful young person equipped to enjoy the good things in life, I fell flat on my face.

In those days enjoying your twenties, from the view I perceived, was a successful college stint, successful drinking, and sports, along with the most prominent, "broad jumping", or fucking as a sport, if you will.

Looking back that seems so simple. And with the creative and manipulative mind I had, I could have probably done well in all of those categories. But, I of course needed to punish myself to pay for the sins I committed in my early childhood, which is the way I interpreted my Catholic upbringing.

What comes to mind for me was the time I pissed myself in first grade and the nun shamed me. Look, it was bad enough I pissed myself, but to be put on center stage in front of about twenty of my peers was tough. I'd have to face them the next day, not to mention the next eight years at this school.

Well, by the age of about twenty six I found myself urinating in the middle of the front room carpet of some girl's apartment, who I was dating, while in a drunken stupor. I had been on a heroin and morphine binge for the prior few months straight, when my supply dried up. I had attempted to drown the withdrawals away with heavy alcohol consumption.

I still contend that the toilet was right in front of me when I started to pee. But that didn't go over too well as one could probably imagine. I was awoken to a stern slap in the face. All

I remember is that I was enjoying a well needed pee. I could swear I saw the toilet right in front of me and the flow was going directly into the toilet bowl, and it was so relieving. Well, until the slap in the face along with this woman yelling, "what the f*** are you doing, pissing on my carpet?!"

I remember feeling so violated that someone would interrupt me while enjoying a good pee. And for her to dump me for that? Well I found it to be a bit harsh. Ok, I'm laughing. I guess it could be considered a bit inappropriate and maybe even a deal breaker.

When reality hit me in the face the next morning I realized that my attempt to drown my opiate withdrawal with alcohol doesn't work to well? And thus the results of that night just seemed to be in line with the historical relationship trends throughout my life. Alcohol, drugs, and interpersonal relationships just don't seem to mix very well?

* * * * *

I always did have this uneasy feeling of not fitting in. Regardless of where I was, I just didn't feel 'part of', I felt that I was just an outsider. The effort I put into trying to fit in, use to drain me to the point of exhaustion. I just wanted to feel normal, though it was kind of like a square peg wanting to fit in to a round hole. It just never felt right to me. I don't care if I was in a grocery store line, a party, or even when I was locked up somewhere. I would turn on the chameleon act searching for the role I needed to play to be a part of society.

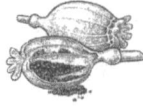

CHAPTER SIX

Life throws a lot of curves which every person walking this earth experiences sometime in their lives. I now see that my responses when encountering the curves over the years were fear based reactions. I had been in fear my entire life for whatever reason, and my actions in response to the curves seemed to have been very poor, to say the least.

My experiences, looking back at the outcome of my ill-advised decisions made during those times, were nothing but knee jerk reactions which led me to find that the curves turned to dead ends. These decisions ultimately forced me to learn the hard way. What I found throughout the years was that I really needed to regroup and take an extended pause in future situations, where I was faced with the need to take action in life. I began to realize that my life depended on it. And I learned some very valuable lessons that led to "wisdom" (which is defined as experience, knowledge, and good judgment). Wisdom is not a given trait, it is rather something that every person has instilled in them as somewhat of a seed with vast potential.

There is definitely something to be said about "learning the hard way". However the outcome of the learning experiences are seemingly all dependent on the willingness to take heed of bad decisions by growing that seed of "wisdom". It took me many years and many, many, horrible consequences for my poor decisions that I ultimately benefited in a strange way, if that's possible? Growth of one's mind can either flourish with wisdom, or be devastated by negativity, thus being darkened by doubt. Never giving up was the route I had to force myself to believe, or I know I would have just been thoroughly defeated in life? It was the "Good Judgment" part that took me so very long to grasp, in growing that seed of wisdom.

After nearly 15 years of continuous and complete insanity, living on the dark side I crashed hard. I began my trek into seeking out that God forbidden heroin rodeo of this world.

I had spent nearly a third of my life locked up in jail on the installment plan, and the rest of the days imprisoned in the life of chaos. I suddenly found myself completely distraught, drained of all of the spiritual, emotional, and psychological energy I ever had. It was time to get help, though it was only due to the court system. I just never could get myself to the point of seeking help. You see, crazy people don't know they're crazy. So why on earth would I solicit help for something that I didn't have a problem with? The only problem I had was, I just couldn't get enough of what I needed' and not even Walgreens had enough of what I wanted.

The straw that finally broke the camel's back, as I look back, was that I had lost so many friends to heroin and other opioid related deaths. And through the years of toiling within

the life of morphine and heroin addiction, I had consumed myself with attempting to rid the grip that opioid addiction had
on me, as not to be just another statistic.

If you go inside the mind of a person addicted to opiates,
you'll find it is a very simple and narrow minded outlook on
daily life. However, it is also a very convoluted and dark style
of mindset. It paints a picture of deceit and manipulation with
one thing in mind, where it is always a means to an end. And
the end is always with them getting what they want and someone else getting screwed.

It goes something like this: It's about 11 am. That their con-
scious mind is beckoned by their monkey. Unless of course
the monkey began to get restless from being under fed the day
before. That all depends upon what part of the roller coaster track they're on. With a junkie there are times that proverbial windfalls are in the stars. Maybe they cashed in an old
life insurance policy, or a 401k that they were never going to
touch. Possibly the one last and final loan from a relative, an
old friend, or a bar owner they knew for years. Perhaps a drug
store they previously robbed that had more narcotics than they
expected to haul in. Or maybe even a girlfriend who recently
got an inheritance? Or, you conned her into cashing in her 401k.
You're most definitely going to pay her back as soon as you get
a settlement of some kind, honest. "I wouldn't lie to you about
something like that, honey!"

Just like "Rosanna Rosanna Danna" would tell you..."It's
always something."

And in all seriousness, with a junkie it is always something. Something they need, to get something they want. They always think they need it. But, truth be told, they just f**** wanted it!

An old friend of mine once told me something I really did not want to hear and even infuriated me. I had stopped by his pharmacy to see if I could just "once more" get another prescription of Percodan to help me with my heroin withdrawals. I swore it would be the last time I would ever step foot in his store again. It was the same old song and dance I had been giving him for about six months. He just looked at me and said, "I'm sorry, I just can't do it". I replied, "Look, I swear it this time! I'm sick as a dog and I'm ready to ween off the stuff". He just replied and said "if you're going to get off the stuff, start right now. Trust me, you're not going to die, even though you might feel like it". And that is the one thing junkies fear the most.

Withdrawal. It's a bitch to say the least. What I always wondered about was, why it is so fearful to a junkie. Some of us could walk into a store loaded with people shopping and stick a gun in the face of a cashier and demand money. It's real uncommon for the police to get there fairly quick and shoot you. Or even a patron of the store to shoot you. We could pierce a needle into our body and inject a possible hot shot, (lethal dose) risking death. But, when it comes to facing withdrawal head on? Pussies. Just like a whimpering little child. "Please, I'm getting sick!" Help me!

The bottom line is, withdrawals just seem to expose every nerve in your body. It's like a train car coming at you full speed, and you feel completely paralyzed, while you anticipate the impact. It sends signals to the brain that say you're absolutely useless and there is no hope, unless...

Unless you invite the beast back into your soul. It gets so very ugly. And it's when you realize that your pet monkey has grown to be an angry gorilla.

The pharmacist I knew was a friend for years, and it was in his home while I was in my teen years that his brother and I found a treasure chest full of pharmaceutical cocaine, morphine, tincture of opium, and Demerol, stashed away in the attic of their home. It's where I originally broke my opiate virginity. Within a month, my friend and I had fallen in love with opiates. And from there, into my twenties I was on what seemed to be a never ending ride in the world of opioids.

It was years later, my pharmacist friend opened his own pharmacy. When I heard about it, I immediately made a visit to see him, with a stolen prescription I wrote, for 120 Percodan.

The look I got from him was priceless. It was a half-smile, half frown, while he shook his head. He just said, *"Nice try, I know Dr. T****'s hand writing, and this my friend is not it."*

However, he did ultimately dispense the 120 Percodan for me, with a verbal disclaimer that it was the last time he'd do it.

Back then, if I saw someone had money or drugs that could help feed my monkey, there was absolutely no way a person could justify not giving it to me.

My pharmacist friend did ultimately fill a plethora of Percodan prescriptions for me, until he ultimately ended up in Federal prison.

It's the moment we junkies need something that counts. We're sick! What the hell else were we supposed to do? (Poor junkie ;)

Ok, now it's ten after eleven and the junkies mind is already past the doom and gloom of yesterday's regrets and guilt. Their eyes now open and its brainstorming time. How the hell am I going to get what I need today?

Now you have to understand that junkies always have at least a few people in their lives. More than likely it's the "man" the dealer. You always know where your "man" is. And if you don't? You are certainly going to make it your business to find him. And you need to know if he has dope, how good it is, how much it is, and last but not least, will he front you just one bag until you get the check you've been waiting for. The one that really doesn't exist. Hell, you have to try.

Then, as you know, misery loves company, and I always had a buddy somewhere. It's not necessarily to get high with them, or even to have someone to talk to. The real reason is, they may have seen 'the man' (Heroin dealer) or know where he is. And they also may just know of a scam of sorts to get some cash?

As far as having another junkie buddy, it's just an extension to get what you want. Two junkies may talk about things of substance, but it's probably only a minute or two after you shoot your dope, and then you're only mumbling words while you're nodding off, which neither party even remembers what the f*** you talked about.

And it is most likely the junkie has a parent, family member, or old friend that the junkie needs when they feel they need a shoulder to cry on. That is if you haven't exhausted all attempts to get something out of them.

Holy shit, it's almost noon! The monkey is beginning to nudge you again, as to say "don't forget me". The junkie begins to think if he has anything left from yesterday. And more times than not the answer is most likely just a bit of powder residue on the packet from the day before. Or, maybe a bit of a wash left in the spoon? Son of a bitch, it's time to get up and begin brainstorming, again. It's so damn taxing.

Hell, its past noon and the junkie knows the shit ain't going to land on the door step. Time to get up, and shower? Hell no. Not unless he's going to go cash a fake prescription for some Dilaudid, Percocet, OxyContin? OxyContin wasn't even around when I was using. Another thing I f*** up! But yes, if you're going to cash a fake prescription you need to look presentable. And while you're in the shower getting ready, you can think of a good story to tell the pharmacist of why you might be needing the stuff anyway.

I remember a time that I took a prescription for sixty 4 mg. Dilaudid (semi synthetic morphine) into a pharmacy to have it filled. When I handed it to the pharmacist I got a raised eyebrow look as would be expected, given I was only about 25 years old. What the hell would a 25 year old guy need with sixty f**** Dilaudid? Well, I told him I just found out I had pancreatic cancer. I didn't even know what the hell the pancreas was at the time, but I had it. He must have felt sorry for me because he had it ready in minutes. I walked out one happy SOB. Hell, I had enough to last me about ten days for purposes of weening off heroin. But, truth be told, I did about thirty the first day. Then I knew I had to conserve. I had to be smart. This was going to be the time that I was going to quit and help bring me to the end stage of my drug use, I thought to myself.

Well, about an hour later I decided to quit after the holidays. Why ruin the holidays, so I did the other thirty in less than two days.

It's not even 2 pm and this junkie is seriously making an attempt to get his rickety ass out of bed. Bones aching, gagging, sniffling, and feeling what you could imagine a 99 year old man may feel. But he knows that he has to find a way to feed the monkey, and when he does he will once again feel like Jesus' son. With that motivation he gets out of bed and begins his trek as if being moved by some strong momentum derived from his will to score his daily fix. I guess one could equate it to a race car driver visualizing the finish line. It's an energy boost with the means to an end. And anyone or anything in his way will be meaningless after he passes them by extracting any worth he can pluck away from them.

By 3pm the junkies mind is honed in on getting whatever he can do to feed the monkey as it tugged away at his soul. There are so many ideas that pop into the junkies head at this point of his venture, as his tongue becomes razor sharp in his quest to obtain what he needs.

An example of my personal recollection of being at this moment in time is this: One day I had finally got my apathetic butt moving by coming up with a scheme that might just get me what I wanted to halt my withdrawals. I stopped at the nearest phone booth and scoured the yellow pages for some nearby doctor's offices. From previous experience the best doctors to hit were smaller mom and pop type of offices. Doctors that practiced internal medicine were commonly the ones who seemed to diagnose and treat a patient in the initial visit. Emergency rooms were ok, but they'd already been bombarded by the common drug seekers. And the fact you'd probably only net about 12 to 15 pills at the visit, unless of course you weren't booted out with some useless muscle relaxer or anti-inflammatory. No, for me, I liked the smaller and out of the way docs who had their own little private practice. It just felt cozier and it always seemed to give an experienced junkie a personal touch where you could work on the emotional and psychological side of the doctor. (So horribly wrong when I think back).

The day that rings so true to form for this deceitful serpent of a human I was then, was when I honed in on a doctor who had his own private practice. It was a doctor who seemingly needed as many new patients as he could get. I made a quick stop into the lobby where the doctor was also his own receptionist. When he greeted me in the front lobby, his warm welcome played right into my despicable game. I said that I was in town for a short period of time and I was experiencing some very bad headaches, and that I could feel one coming on at this very moment. He gave me a clipboard with a new patient form to fill out and invited me into an exam room. He asked me to relax a moment while he discharged a patient he had in another room.

The moment he exited the room to see to his other patient, I began to rifle through the drawers for any possible drugs or more importantly some blank prescription pads. If the prescription pads already had the doctors DEA NUMBER (identification number required when filling a prescription for a scheduled drug) which were almost like gold. Sure enough there was a pad in a drawer which I tore off about five and slipped them into my pocket.

Moments later the doctor entered the room to examine me and he asked me to explain my symptoms and describe my pain level. As I explained my symptoms which I experienced an aura coming whereas I felt dizzy, nausea, and a sense of confusion setting in. I went on to say that this had always been a precursor to horrible migraine headaches I experienced almost every couple of weeks. I mentioned that I had been previously prescribed a drug called 'Ergot' (medication that narrows the blood vessels) and 'Percodan' (synthetic morphine). I told him the combination of the two drugs were the only thing that alleviated my horrible pain. And I mentioned that the symptoms were rapidly coming on that very moment. The doctor led me into another examination room where he asked me to rest a few moments with the lights off, and he'd be back soon.

I must mention that I have had years of experience in describing many different pain related symptoms. It came from years of training I underwent from my pharmacist friend, a gynecologist friend, and other junkies.

Shortly after I had rested in the room, which I felt slight withdrawals begin to manifest within my body, the doctor came to discuss his recommendations. He first asked where I was from, what brought me to Milwaukee, and asked what I did for a living. As I lay on the exam table with this doctor sitting beside me, lights off, and the door opened a crack for minimal light, I told him my story. And a completely outlandish story, I began to tell him. I said that I was on the Cleveland Indians minor league baseball team which I played third base. And our team was in Wisconsin for a week of training and playing. Now who could come up with such an extraordinary story, other than this insane junkie I was. Now either this doctor believed me, or he figured I was completely insane, but he pulled out his prescription pad while saying that he would write a onetime script for 30 'Percodan' and 12 'Ergot'. He told me to rest in the dark room a bit before I left, as to hopefully relieve the pain. Needless to say I didn't lay there long before paying the $30 doctor bill and hightailing out of that office.

Now it is about 5 pm and this junkies on his way to finish his day's work. I had in fact worked at many different jobs over the years, and I guess you could say it was like I just finished work. I completed the day's work by going to the nearest pharmacy to fill my prescriptions. Now the nearest pharmacy to this doctor's office was important because the pharmacist would no doubt know this physicians hand writing. And that would lend credibility to the authenticity of the prescription, so the pharmacist would likely fill it without feeling the need to call the doctor to verify it. The reason this was important in the scheme of things was for the fact I still had about five blank prescriptions I had pilfered from the doctor's office. It's bad enough I conned this poor guy out of narcotics, but I totally violated him further by stealing his prescriptions. How despicable when I look back.

Having some blank prescriptions gave me a good chance to replicate the script by forging it with the same dispensing instructions and as close as I could get to his handwriting.

Some facts about my history was that I had years of practice in forging my mother's signature back when I had absentee permission slips in my high school days. And I also studied Latin at the nearby libraries to understand the prescription instructions that doctors wrote when giving a script.

* * * * *

Looking back I see what a waste I made of my life. I guess you could say that for someone to go to these lengths to get what I wanted back then, it also says what I might have accomplished by walking the path of academics and doing the right thing. What an insane and twisted way to live.

* * * * *

When I had written the duplicate prescriptions of my original, I could have it filled at other pharmacies. So, back then if the pharmacy questioned the authenticity of the prescription, they could call the doctor to verify it was legitimate. And if I saw the pharmacist call the doctor, I knew it was the last duplicate I could render without having the police come walking in the store. There were times I was able to duplicate as many as ten times on one prescription. That's ten times the amount of narcotics. But, as the old saying in many twelve step programs tell you, "one is too many, and a thousand never enough".

Well it's about 7pm, and the junkie is back to a nearby shooting gallery. For me the gallery was anywhere I had laid my head that night. I stayed in basements, ones where I knew the people and sometimes I even found an apartment building with an unlocked lobby and slipped down to the locker area or laundry room. If it had running water it was a plus, if not, I'd stop by a gas station and fill a bottle with water. I'd need the water to soak down the Percodan. If I had 30 Percodan, I would soak them down, and I'd inject them all in one sitting. And like I mentioned about what the twelve step people said in that "a thousand was never enough"? If I had as many as 300, I'd soak them down, and I went until I nodded off into 'Percodan Land'. It's just what I did in those days. Complete insanity to put it lightly.

* * * * *

By 10 pm the junkie is nodding off, if they're fortunate (in a junkies world, fortunate, meant you had a good day of gathering) I wish I could tell you the entire process of addiction was all so horrifying. But I must say that the feeling from heroin or opiates was phenomenal to put it lightly. I'd be lying if I said it didn't. You've probably heard that old saying of "feeling like Jesus Son"? Well...I'll leave it at that.

But, as reality sets in at about 2 o'clock in the morning, the time most "normal" people are in bed resting, this junkie would be awoken by his monkey. Even that monkey was spoiled when there were fortuitous days of gathering a big stash. This f***** thing (the monkey) would want to stuff itself with more. That monkey is the one that says a thousand is never enough. You probably couldn't find a poppy field that would yield enough for this monkey I carried around during the times of my using. You'd think it were a full grown gorilla at times. Gluttonous thing it surely is.

And, so now that you probably have an idea of what a crazy time it can be in the day of the life of a junkie. You be the judge of whether it's easy. Truth be told, it's one crazy day. And just when you swear you'll never live another day in that lifestyle, you wake up scheming about where your fix is coming from the next. It's a never ending vicious cycle. Every time you think you're out...it pulls you back in.

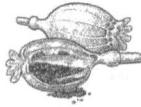

CHAPTER SEVEN

In reality, the life of a junkie rarely goes smooth, or consistent, if you dare choose to use the word "consistent". It's such a roller coaster that the only "consistent" thing about addiction is that the monkey will stay by your side as long as you allow it to.

Before you know it, each and every day will begin with one eye over your shoulder. You know that you have alienated someone, somewhere, somehow. It's just what happens while living on the dark side of life. And in that dark side of life, you become captive in a virtual hell on earth.

Recovery for a junkie begins with the first day clean, and continues day to day, though the moods and attitudes toward life swing like a pendulum. And, make no mistake about it, the first few days, if not longer, go minute by minute like a dripping faucet that will not stop no matter what you do. Believe me, it is torture beyond anything imaginable. At least it feels that way.

The good is that it will subside, and eventually go away. The bad is that you just cannot see a possible end while suffering through it. That monkey will do it's best to convince you there is no possibility of feeling better without feeding it.

One thing that really gets that monkey riled up is when you've quit long enough to have accumulated the least bit of money. Holy shit does that monkey shake your cage. And if your cage is open, so to speak, if you're not locked up somewhere that is, it is almost too inviting. Your mind races from zero to sixty in seconds flat. And that horrible tug of war in your mind begins. Even if you're at the point where the physical withdrawals have passed, the urging of the monkey will tell you "your bones still ache, don't they? Sure they do". "Remember that you still can't sleep well" and it's just about then that you yawn, big and wide. "It'll take that away too!" Then you just might remember that smell of the dope being cooked up in the spoon. You know, that vinegary smell that almost made you gage just by the very whiff of it?

Well, I sincerely hope most people reading this, have not experienced any of this insanity, and pray they never will.

* * * * *

One school of thought in respect to withdrawal from heroin and other opioids I found to be interesting, was that I saw it affected people in very different ways. For me it was that once heroin was eliminated, the physical withdrawals were much the same as what seemed to be the norm for most all people. There is the common sequence of physical symptoms that cycle in the human body while the drug is cleansed from the system. Most of the physical symptoms are very much dependent on the length of time the person used, and the amounts that were used, which determine the severity of the symptoms.

But, the one other factor that I find extremely perplexing in the elimination of heroin and other opiates from the individual is what uniquely varies from person to person. What is so very different in the psychological process of withdrawal is what can also determine the relapse probability. This is where I see the various Twelve Step programs almost a necessity for a majority of people.

Herein lies some different scenarios that vary from person to person.

One scenario is that of the addict who was afflicted with troubling personality traits prior to using heroin. There are many people that can have psychological hang ups which many times precede ever using drugs. Whether it's troubling family history and upbringing, individual mistakes haunting the person due to poor decision making prior to using, or just plain boredom. And many times it's just the lack of productivity because of procrastination, which in lies a whole different defect of character.

The bottom line is what I contend to be another aspect which heroin and other drugs in the opiate family, is that the unstated properties are the ones that are uniquely masked.

When a person uses heroin, it not only numbs physical pain, but it very uniquely diminishes the state of any unsettling psychological issues. I'm telling you, this stuff is so very cunning and baffling.

The horrible part of the withdrawal stage is that not only will you experience the common physical symptoms, not to mention any aches or pain from previous injuries. Then, what adds insult to injury is that the worries, anxiety, and guilt that were present before drowning it with heroin, come back in what can be likened to light speed, and it hits tenfold. After mulling it over in my mind, I guess the only way I can attempt to describe it, is this scenario; a man born to wealth who never experienced anything but pampering from the time he's born, suddenly wakes up one day with malnutrition living in a desert with no food or water, though his mindset stayed with him. If he could find a gun he'd surely blow his brains out. Weird scenario? Probably. But truth be told, its hell on earth in a matter of three long days.

There you are back to square one, with the snowballing effect of the additional guilt and shame from the previous day. It's a completely disastrous feeling, like being hit with a brick. And the only thing that can take it away is...of course...more heroin. It's a vicious cycle that is next to impossible to break without some type of intervention. Whether it's family intervention, relationship collapse, court troubles, or even tragedies of health impairment due to the usage. And for most addicts, it's not until then do they come to the realization that the gig may be up. And even then it seems as though the addicts very next thought is "ok, one more fix for the road." Once again they will swear that one last time will be it. And deep inside that afflicted, sick mind, they themselves may just believe it.

But in reality, it's all a big lie like everything else in their lives during these times. I truly wish I could say that there is much hope, though it's for the very few that it is possible.

It's just a big bowl of mixed chaos, but amidst all of the insanity of this lifestyle, there may just be the seed, which could be the one saving grace and secret to success. Just as the Poppy Seed looms over mankind searching for its next victim, therein lies a glimpse of hope that may just help to eradicate the grip opioids have on your life. It all depends on the individual.

Inside the voluminous amount of chaotic troubles that surface during an internal intervention within the mind of a junkie, there always seems to be one fact that cannot be ignored. It's the certainty that your life has become completely unmanageable. And the one saving grace may just be, that you gave your logic a voice in the matter of the facts surrounding your downfall.

Maybe it was that faint whisper of something a loved one said, which triggered enough guilt along with common sense that hit a nerve. And the nerve may have been hit just right that you couldn't drown it no matter how hard you tried.

For me, it was a moment in time that I recall hearing my mother's voice, while I was at the height of my addiction. It's something I will always remember and never will forget. She came to visit me at Froedtert Memorial hospital, in Milwaukee, while I was shackled to a hospital bed and under police guard. I had my second bout of endocarditis (infection around the outer sack of the heart) and I clearly remember her looking down at me with tears in her eyes. She reached over toward me and said "Every time you put a needle in your arm, you put a needle in my heart "and she began to weep. All I could think of was this big syringe, with a big, long needle, piercing her heart. Hell of a way to ruin my drug usage. "Way to go mom".

In all seriousness it was a very gut wrenching moment which alerted my mind to the fact that I was not only hurting myself, I was in fact affecting so many other people. Again, I had been so self-centered and selfish.

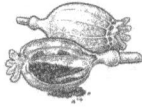

CHAPTER EIGHT

Just as the little poppy seed grew to become the infamous dream catcher, it has captured and destroyed so many lives.

And so I present to you the darkest circle of turmoil known to mankind. It's called *heroin*, one of Mr. Opium's offspring.

And from that little seed, the addict too grows so similar in the way of seemingly an innocent little taste of fun and promises of ecstasy through emotional escape.

One thing I will admit is that heroin is all of what is likely described by many of the famous names that have used it. And I cannot deny that I sometimes daydream about just being able to once more do a hit, just one! It was such a passionate love affair of mine, that the thought of the just one more may always enter my mind.

However, given all the living hell that goes along with the lifestyle that I now am completely well versed on, I just refuse to take that first drop of alcohol, the temptation of one hit of morphine or heroin. This is mainly because throughout the many years of fighting the very urge of it, I found a natural bliss. A bliss that was right in front of me all along. It's called the ultimate appreciation of the life I was given. And being grateful for each and every breath I take is beyond the wonderment of joy. And it's the love and appreciation of the people in my life today, that I find my pleasure.

Life can be difficult enough without recreational substance use as a form of pleasure. Adding substances to enhance relaxation or to fine tune ones social skills, goes completely against the human ability to develop our true and natural capabilities.

Our world nowadays has become so much of a quest for ease and self-satisfaction that we seemed to have slowly become a "ME" society. "ME" as in My Egoism, as opposed to My Endowment.

* * * * *

In my experience, I'd have to say the word 'ME' defines 'My Enemy', as I have always been my worst enemy.

Thirty some years ago I swore to completely eliminate opioids from my life, due to the never ending thirst I had for them, along with the years of pain and suffering it took to quit.

At about 20 years into recovery, I had an umbilical hernia surgery with mesh, which supposedly makes the pain of healing more difficult. At the time I was fearful of the very thought of using opioids of any kind, that I flushed a full prescription without even taking one tablet. I just literally rolled around in pain and deferred to crying and moaning just to avoid the possibility of falling in love with opioids all over again. I loved them that much.

In reality, opioids truly are a Godsend, and they definitely have their place in the medical profession, as surely as antibiotics do. Opiates are also one of the best tools in the realm of compassionate care of pain and suffering. What gave opioids a bad name are guys like myself, whose brains get in the way of desecrating the good name they should carry.

I know it is a big bowl of chaos and confusion for the medical professionals in their attempts to compassionately treat pain while avoiding the future pain of addiction. I get that. But, now we see the huge gap between the tight regulations of opioids versus the compassionate treatment of pain. On one hand physicians are told to be more attentive to the voice of the patient who is in pain. And on the other, physicians are accused of overprescribing opioids. The medical professionals now find themselves in a quandary whereas if they listen to the voice of their patient and do in fact treat pain which they deem appropriate, they may find that they're accused of overprescribing. On the contrary a physician may find themselves being blamed for being too stringent and unsympathetic of a patient's cry for pain relief.

* * * * *

The truth about opioid abuse in our country is fueled by so many different things, which makes it so difficult for medical professionals to get their arms around.

First of all, we have heroin abuse, which is probably the most prominent issue that concerns people, due to the stigma that goes with it. Heroin addiction is a dirty, filthy, and dangerous habit. For one, street heroin's make up is a big variety of whatever the hell is in the ingredients, beside actual heroin. And day to day no one really knows what the street stuff is going to be mixed with. The main factor that leads to the overdoses seen in emergency rooms, and in the morgues, are most times due to the substances used in diluting the heroin sold on the streets.

Fentanyl is what seems to be the most notable thing found in the heroin nowadays. Fentanyl is a very powerful opioid derivative painkiller that is 50 to 100 times more powerful than morphine, with a very rapid onset and short life duration which can certainly account for the overdose, not to mention that its low cost shows more profit for dealers.

The heroin we see on the streets in our country nowadays comes through a variety of avenues, which makes its way to the end users. If you look at the heroin trade from the local street level it seems that it hasn't changed much since when I was using it, which was over 30 years ago.

From what I see and hear now it's the same old stuff, with the exception that it's said to be cheaper and more potent.

I remember a time that a buddy and I were hurting because the streets were seemingly dried up of available heroin. We heard through the grapevine that someone was coming in from Mexico with some good black tar heroin. So, as the adamant addicts we were then, whereas our whole world was consumed with the hunt and kill of heroin, we made sure we were in the front of the line to get some. We sat at some old neighborhood home on the near south side of Milwaukee waiting for the person to arrive with it. There were about six Spanish speaking people in the house, some of them women and children. With the anticipation growing, our nerves on end, and our monkeys digging their claws into our souls, we waited. Now we didn't speak Spanish, so it was difficult trying to get a clear picture of just how long we'd have to wait. In an attempt to get the attention of the guy who was getting it for us, we pointed at our watch and said we needed to head out to get some elsewhere. Truth be told we didn't have anyone else that we could get any from, but we needed to give the impression that it wouldn't be a problem going elsewhere.

Our contact just kept telling us to wait a bit longer, the best he could in English. He kept pointing at the other room and motioned to wait. Well, if the stuff was coming soon there was actually no way we were leaving.

As it turned out, there was a woman who was already in the house that had just come in from Mexico. Well, she was doing her best to shut out the balloons full of heroin, she brought in with her. Apparently the guy we knew was waiting for her to get it out, sift through the shit, clean off the balloons and extract the heroin out. And yes, I admit that we found it to be acceptable, given how desperate we were. Boy, you talk about a shitty deal?

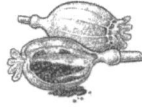

CHAPTER NINE

Now Afghanistan is the main producer of opium which is exported to other countries, where it is then processed into heroin and morphine. Remember, our military is guarding the poppy fields in Afghanistan, so for the life of me I can't understand how it gets out of the country.

Opium is one of the biggest cash cows known to man, and has been for centuries, throughout the entire world.

The heroin industry is an empire that produces nothing but a strain on every facet of society's mere existence. If you sit down and think of the domino effect heroin and opioid addiction cause, it's mind boggling to say the least.

If we take a Birdseye view of this epidemic in our country, you will see the poor mixed up souls destroying themselves. And though they may just seem to be the hopeless deplorable addicts of our society, they are also someone's sons, daughters, mothers, fathers, and loved ones.

The very sad truth of this epidemic is that we see the overcrowded jails and institutions, the strain on the court system, and the insurmountable financial strain it puts on all of us.

I would suggest that to really comprehend the actual devastation it causes, would be by looking at it in the following sequence; the heroin trade is an under the radar sale which produces absolutely no revenue for governments in the way of tariffs or taxes. The industry's sales force shows no income, so that is pure profit for each hand that touches it.

Federal law enforcement agencies hunt down the (heroin) industry's importers and sales people. Local police in turn spend endless hours pursuing the crimes committed by the users. Then you have our judicial system, whose resources are already taxed, now facing overcrowded jails and prisons, due to drug related crimes. Now we have the financial burden of the court appointed legal defense and incarceration costs which are astronomical.

The state probation and parole boards then become overwhelmed by the amount of people under supervision for drug related crimes, adding more costs, along with drug screening charges from the labs. Some are referred to other agencies specializing in drug rehabilitation that the users are referred to, which the costs are astronomical.

Then you have our healthcare system flooded with drug users and low end dealers attempting to obtain pharmaceutical opioids from doctors, for purposes of an alternative to heroin. We also have the health related ailments that come with it, such as heart disease, hepatitis C, AIDS, infectious pestilence, and for some death. All which creates a domino effect on their families in the way of hurt, shame, guilt, and depression.

There is now a family member needing anti-depressants, due to the stress of watching their addicted loved one, adding more burden to families and additional healthcare costs. There's the spouse and children that the user can no longer afford to care for, who unfortunately end up on social welfare programs, social security, and food stamps. And the domino effect goes on down the line, even touching people who had nothing to do with any part of the equation, though every aspect of their healthcare costs, taxes, and insurance go up because of the epidemic.

I know I'm getting dramatic, but I think you get my point on just how devastating this stuff really is.

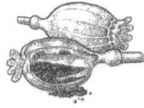

CHAPTER TEN

Now I know that it's a tall task in getting our arms around this epidemic, but the programs suggested by the existence of other countries attempting to get a handle on it, should lend some credence. Just the fact of less crime, healthcare issues, and judicial strain, should be enough to give it a try.

England's heroin addiction statistics have recently shown a 79% decline over the past decade. There a number of factors that have contributed to this decline which are availability, the aging of a large group of the previous "drug generation" people, and the criminal justice laws in England.

When a heroin addict seeks or is referred to their drug treatment program they are given a dose of heroin daily and sent home. They are also assisted with rehabilitation efforts such as housing, employment, and counseling. Sound crazy? Maybe, but they appear to be having better luck than in our country.

England took heed of a program that had begun in Zurich, Switzerland. It was originally set up by the advice of a prominent researcher, Ambros Uchtenhagen, a professor of Psychiatry at Zurich University. There had been an area of Zurich prior to the program taking off, which was deemed the largest open drug park known to society. It was known as an open pit of heroin addicts lying passed out in their own blood, urine, and feces, and even some of them dead from overdose.

After 30 days of the Zurich heroin treatment program being opened, drug related crime dropped over 60%. This is a stark reality of the heroin and opioid epidemic throughout the entire world.

Even though the idea of implementing a "Heroin Treatment Program" in the United States may seem counterintuitive, I contend that it may just be a viable option that needs more attention in our country. It's proven to take away most of the criminal aspect that runs parallel with opioid addiction. And, just think of the strain it puts on our healthcare system, filled with drug seekers, overdoses, not to mention sepsis, hepatitis, and other health related factors. It is voluminously mind boggling when you think about it.

As for pharmaceutical opioid abusers, it's basically the same hunt and kill process that heroin addicts consume themselves with. I would contend that the vast majority of pharmaceutical opioid abusers began by recreational use of either Percocet or Vicodin, or had already been accustomed to heroin abuse. Since it's a proven fact of knowing exactly what you're getting with pharmaceutical opioids, many users prefer that, rather than shuffling through the heroin world. When people are chasing down doctors for opioid prescriptions it's because they know what they are getting, as opposed to heroin and other street drugs. And, it also does not seem to carry with it the stigma that heroin addiction does; whereas pharmaceutical addicts can point to the fact that they are at least not a filthy, deplorable, junkie, in some back alley injecting heroin.

The problem with pharmaceutical drugs is that it's very definition comes from the Latin word pharmakeia, which carries the meaning of "sorcery" or "witchcraft", and that kind of says it all.

I neither profess that I have a clue of what the correlation between drugs being developed for cure, or even the ones for pain, have to do with sorcery, but my point is, that to me, it says abuse of drugs become sorcery of sorts. Yes, that's kind of deep and even weird for some junkie to give a sermon on drug abuse, but the fact is that the very existence of opium poppies are further evidence that it is the "god of pain" . And perhaps man made drugs are false gods? I'm laughing, because I have no clue what the whole religious interpretation of this stuff has to do with addiction. However, I can tell you that my personal real life experience with heroin, other opioids and especially Methadone (manmade) they do in fact have very differing withdrawal symptoms. My experience with Methadone were perhaps the worst withdrawals of any addictive drug, i.e. Percodan / Percocet (Oxycodone), Dilaudid, (Hydromorphone) codeine, and especially heroin.

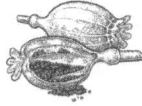

CHAPTER ELEVEN

I n 2001, there was a Joint Commission report on "Federal Guidelines for Opioid Treatment Programs" which is 82 pages long. (The Joint Commission is a United States-based nonprofit tax-exempt organization that accredits more than 21,000 health care organizations and programs in the United States. There is also an international branch that accredits medical services around the world. A majority of state governments recognize Joint Commission accreditation as a condition of licensure and the receipt of Medicaid and Medicare reimbursements. The Joint Commission is based in the Chicago suburb of Oakbrook Terrace, Illinois).

Within the guidelines published by the "Joint Commission" there is another 358 page guideline from SAMHSA (Substance Abuse and Mental Health Services Administration) and those guidelines dictate, or suggest, as they say, how opioid addiction treatment needs to be handled. Yes, 358 pages of the "how to" treat opioid addicts with one of the worst drugs known to man, "Methadone".

In my opinion, which I can tell you by way of firsthand experience, is that Methadone dependency has to be one of the worse drugs to detoxify from the human body. The withdrawal from Methadone can last months due to the chemical makeup of this drug, which wreaks havoc within the nervous system. It's absolutely insane.

However, it does create jobs within government funded programs and it is justified by showing statistics of criminal decline within in patient caseload. It also supplies our government with known drug abusers, ultimately having records of its registered constituents. Does our government keep files on registered drug abusers? Hell, I don't know. It does however give them justification for agencies such as all of the organizations I have mentioned, and more.

Granted, Methadone maintenance programs do give the appearance that they are taking control of the misuse factors associated with heroin and other opiates. One major factor that has become a strong selling point for justifying these clinics, is that the criminal statistics which accompany the abuse of these drugs will no doubt show success when analyzing the patient population at these clinics, prior to treatment.

Do you think that the drug companies don't benefit from pushing more and more opioid concoctions out to the public, only to once again benefit when a person is admitted to a Methadone maintenance program? It's brilliant when you think about it. It keeps the circle of drug dependency going around, and around. I'm willing to bet that the success rate of people getting off Methadone is way lower than actual heroin abusers getting clean.

Then again, I guess we could just go back to what Nancy Reagan said, "Just say no". How did that go over?

In experiencing withdrawal from Methadone, it was seemingly a never ending horrific nightmare. Granted, I was abruptly removed from a two year habit of 80 plus mg. of Methadone and locked in a small infirmary jail cell for almost 20 days.

I can tell you that it was, hands down, the most horrific experience of my entire life.

I literally found myself with visual and auditory hallucinations, where I swore I heard my 18 month old child crying, and while I got up to tend to him, I was awoken by cracking my head on the prison cell door. To add insult to injury, immediately after being awoken by hitting my head, I grabbed a kit Kat bar on my way back to my metal bed, unwrapped it, and bit into it, only to find it was in reality, an ivory soap bar.

You talk about nasty withdrawal symptoms. One positive thing that came from my experience with Methadone, is that I can honestly say that it was the end of my career with opioid dependency.

The complete withdrawal process from Methadone seemed to last for about six months. I can tell you that the first two weeks were literally without sleep. I literally went the first eight days sleepless, with stomach cramps, nausea, tremors, and emotional collapse. There was also a feeling I can only describe as though my nervous system was plugged into a high voltage outlet.

There is definitely something very different in the withdrawal process with Methadone as opposed to heroin.

The contradistinction between the two is the chemistry makeup in which they both possess contrarily. With heroin there is a chemical process that is performed when processing the opium to the end state, of which heroin is produced. Methadone on the other hand, is a completely synthetic drug contrived of manmade chemicals. It was originally developed in Germany by the direction of Adolf Hitler to keep Germany independent from the influence of other countries. For me, the very fact that it was developed under any part of Hitler's rule says to me that its very existence is tainted with an evil core.

Heroin withdrawal is no picnic, I assure you. However, I can tell you that despite the fact that while going through the process of withdrawal from heroin makes you feel like you're going to die, though it is much less taxing on the body. And the elimination of the chemical damage that occurs in a person's body from heroin abuse is very minimal, in comparison to Methadone.

If we look at the epidemic in the United States today, heroin has taken more lives than automobile accidents. That is the horrific reality that we face with the majority of the deaths caused by the strength of the heroin, and also the chemicals that are found in the mixtures of the drugs sold on the streets, namely Fentanyl.

And, if you look at the day in the life of an opioid addict, as I mentioned earlier, it tells of a crazy almost insane addiction in itself. It's the hunt and capture of this daily routine that accompanies this lifestyle. So, as we look at the heroin programs in other countries, as well as Methadone clinics (as much as I hate this drug) these programs do assist in pulling the addict out of the insane daily routine, thus diminishing the criminal acts that accompany this lifestyle.

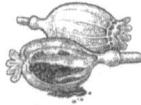

CHAPTER TWELVE

If anyone reading this thinks I am implying that I have an answer for fixing the heroin and opioid abuse problem, forget about it. As for me, you could say it was an act of God intervening in my life to get off the opioid abuse merry go round. It took a few very close encounters with death, irreparable damage to my physical health, and numerous court interventions.

So, as for me giving a speech on how to get off the shit, no. But, what I can offer are some suggestions on how to stay off it. For me it is a twelve step program. Hands down it's the only thing that kept me clean and...I want to say sane, though anyone reading this may question that part. But I am clean, and that is the first step that allows the rest to unfold for me, sometimes quickly, and sometimes slowly, but it does work.

As for suggestions that I believe may help people, there are a few things that I think may be very crucial in having a better understanding of opioid addiction.

There are numerous factors that need to be considered when determining the root cause of each individual case of patients that abuse opioids. First of all, it is my opinion that there is a big difference between addiction and dependency.

There have been numerous times over the years I've heard people pose the question, "how does anyone know if they have an addictive personality?" Honestly it's very difficult to gauge whether someone has an addictive personality from the outside looking in. However, if it is a person that you are close to and have frequent contact with, there are many signs that will alert you to the fact there are definitely obvious traits.

I believe every person walking this earth has their own little pleasures in life that they deeply cherish. This in no way points to the person being an addict or alcoholic.

However, as for a person like myself, I don't just stop at some magic number or hit the proverbial wall of contentment. I take these pleasures way beyond the routine. I drag these pleasures to the extreme. If it's just that my little moments of relaxation on the same old chair, myself, having the addictive personality that I do, I find it very difficult to get up for a phone call, a knock at the door, or to greet a loved one as they come in the room. I want my pleasure. I don't want interruptions of any kind. I just want what I want and I guess you could say that I'm self-absorbed to the nth degree. I don't want interference from anyone or anything. It's about me.

For me, if it were the cold beer, a glass of wine, or marijuana, I was never satisfied with just one. I just always went until I was out cold. It seems that the routine becomes excessive self-absorbency. It seems to go from relaxation to escapism.

It's the person, such as myself, that goes to a bar, a party, or any other type of social gathering and drinks that beer, wine, or drug of choice, and it doesn't stop at the point of social fun and relaxation. It becomes an endless pursuit of complete inebriation. There are no limits. One sign I've seen in myself and a few others, is that I became the person that had indulged to the point of excessive pleasure. Then I found myself setting limits for the next time. And the next time becomes, well... the next time, again. Just one more.

Now, a person that finds themselves setting limits in their future planned use of alcohol or drug of choice, due to prior failures in self-control, would definitely raise a red flag, or should. Some of us just have little self-control when it comes to our pleasures. This I would say, is a problem.

For some it may just be a situational time in one's life that relationship issues of some sort become difficult to the point of feeling the need of temporary escape. That is not a real unusual situation, unless of course you're like me. I found myself creating relationship problems just so I could drink and drug, thus making it a habitual problem. And this problem, becomes THE problem. It's called an addiction.

What makes the whole investigative process into who has an addictive personality so very difficult, is one simple fact, it's the "Human Condition". You just never know, there is no real test whether it's a psychological test, blood panel, or even a

DNA evaluation of one's makeup that definitively tells you that you are in fact an addict.

One thing we do know for sure is this; understanding that we all have what is commonly called that "Human Condition" which says that each and every one of us is vulnerable to its trap.

Another fact is that if we do avoid the known physically addictive substances for recreational pleasures such as alcohol, sedatives, opiates, and even marijuana, we have a hell of a better chance of steering clear of the known pitfall called addiction.

There are much healthier habits to lean toward in life, which can be reading, writing, exercise, and sports. I can tell you that I've never heard of a person lying, cheating, or stealing, in their pursuit of reading, writing, or physical exercise. Ok, maybe in physical exercise, I've cheated.

Opiate dependency most time comes with a person who is a long-term patient of opiates due to an injury, which is also a very different scenario. But that also depends on the history of the patient. What I've seen in observing a number of people who had suffered injuries that warranted long term opioid managed care, varied considerably.

Simply put, it is that with the dependent person, they may just need to be weaned off opioids to avoid abrupt withdrawal. Abruptly stopping the drugs in a patient that had been treated with opioids for six months or more, is likely that they will experience an enhanced pain, precisely where the sustained injury originated. It's just the fact of when long term opioid use is being halted, that will tell if the pain in the affected area is actually healed. The healing process is most commonly when the worst of the actual pain is present. And the withdrawal from opioids in itself, can also magnify any pain that had been masked for so long.

Granted, when I said "simply put" in describing the need to ween a dependent patient from opioids, I didn't mean it would be easy. However, my point is that the difference between an addict being treated by long term opioid care, and the "normal person" who became dependent, under similar circumstances, vastly differs in the realm of treatment, in my opinion. I believe you will find that the "normal" patient, so to speak, will come off the opioid treatment with a much different outlook, while returning to their "normal" lifestyle.

These (normal people) are commonly people who in general have been living that "normal life" so to speak, whereas they have common routines built in to their daily lives. The person who lives a life guided by their regimen of basic habits of sleep, diet, work, leisure activities, and exercise. I guess I could describe "these people" as the neighbors I see leaving for work basically the same time each day, and returning with the same routine. Lights out at the same basic time. Saturday they golf, mow the lawn, or go to the kid's soccer games.

In my description of these people, I no doubt sound like "Gladys Kravitz" from the series "Bewitched" in that I'm a "nosy Parker". Well, truth be told, after many years of insanity within my own head, and living a completely dysfunctional lifestyle, where there seemed to be no rhyme or reason to the lifestyle I led, I felt that I needed to take heed of just how the "normal people" lived. I desperately wanted to know what the other half, so to speak, did the things they did, in my attempt to at least try to be normal. I did learn a lot from just watching these "normal people" and tried to emulate them the best way I could, and then maybe, I thought, I could be the kind of guy who had that one or two evening cocktails. The guy who could have a regular activity or exercise routine. And the same type of guy who would follow the directions on a prescription pill bottle. Well, needless to say I just wasn't that guy, regardless of how hard I tried. I guess you could say that when depicting an "at risk" person, I'd be considered the "red flag" kind of patient, were I to be injured badly enough to warrant pain meds. Me? Forget about it. I'd have the first bottle of 60 Percocet gone in a very short period of time. Screw the directions, and screw the "may be habit forming" warnings. That's a given.

So, on the contrary, an "addicted person" as opposed to the "dependent person" needs to be treated beyond the point of a normal recovery from such an injury. I found that a type of patient with an "addictive personality" like myself, under alike circumstances of recovery from a similar injury, simply couldn't stop obsessing over the fact that they (addictive personality types) needed more opioid managed care, stating the pain still existed. This is where I believe you will find the "at risk" patient resides.

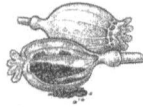

CHAPTER THIRTEEN

I t's the unbalanced life within the "at risk" persons who seem to channel their mind to the easier, softer, way of escape, especially after months of painkillers. The opioids not only masked the said pain, but it also gave the patient a reprieve from a possible psychological uneasiness that existed prior to the injury. This certainly must sound cruel in the way I describe it, however I believe that you would find it to be very accurate if you assessed a number of patients that had been on long term opioid managed care. What better mask could you find than opioids to rid yourself of any and all pain that may exist? That is the "good" and "evil" that just is the plain fact of opioids. They're killers, my friend.

When we speak of heroin addiction for example, we are talking about a whole different animal, so to speak. We are talking about a person who went to the depths of using heroin in the first place. And most times, this is also a person that may go to the extreme of using needles. And with heroin abuse in itself, it is something that definitely says that there are other areas of concern within someone's life that took them to that point in the first place. To even entertain the idea of using heroin as a pastime is definitely a dark space for a person to be in, not to mention the very thought of using a needle as the tool for the presumed pleasure. It is a dark and treacherous venue.

It's very easy to detect an abuser who uses needles, that's a given. However, our society has lent itself to accept pill popping to the extent of being somewhat normal, in that it can be equated with depression, pain, health and wellbeing. Even smoking is an acceptable evil that is considered common and somewhat harmless.

It's the stigma of using needles in drug abuse cases that definitely raises a red flag and labels this person as a deplorable, and rightfully so. The very fact that a person would go to the extreme of needle use, points to a much deeper affliction. The drug abuser who uses needles in their ritual of administering a high, not only points to recklessness in risking disease and infection, it also seems to detect a very self-destructive personality trait, this person displays.

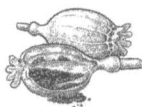

CHAPTER FOURTEEN

There were and still are many different schools of thought on opioid use and addiction. Number one is that opioids are by far the best pain relievers known to mankind. There's obviously proof that opium itself has been the most popular substance since as far back as ancient Egypt. There is proof of this given the fact that the opium poppy pods have been discovered etched in stone in the pyramids. And who knows how far back before then that it became almost a "god" of sorts. There's a reason "Morphine" had been named after "Morpheus" (The god of dreams) should tell you something.

For all we know, the three wise guys may have had opium along with the gold, frankincense, and myrrh, when they went to visit Joseph, Mary, and baby Jesus. Ok, I'm kidding. Bad joke.

In my research of the opioid phenomenon, I found that it is by far the only substance that can contain and relieve physical pain the way opiates do. Not to mention the emotional and psychological relief opioids give. This I know from my own firsthand experience with just about every opiate and opioid derivative there is. Even the copycat drugs that were developed to imitate the opioid affect, have all been proven to be physically addictive. I.e. Methadone, and similar type drugs.

The bottom line is that you just can't beat good old opium and its byproducts, mainly heroin and morphine. Why else would the medical professionals deem it a god from the beginning of their research and trials? And it also tells you why drug companies have been racking their brains for almost a century in an attempt to copy the effects, without the physically addictive characteristics. And just when they think they have something good, it turns out that it too is physically addicting. It's not much different than what was in the early 1800's. Back then, one medical professional thought he had made a groundbreaking discovery. He recognized heroin as being a cure to morphine addiction. We all know how that worked.

It seems that when the drug companies do their best to match opioids magic pain relieving characteristics, with a non-addictive substitute and see their best is not good enough, they settle. Then you see the influx of drug company's sales reps doing their damnedest to get buy-in from the doctors.

You see all kinds of shit pain relievers that are being pushed out there. And the sole reason is to avoid the addiction nightmares in patients. Thus lawsuits and all kinds of legal ramifications. And the bottom line is, as I've always said, and history itself has said, you just can't beat opioids for physical pain.

I'm still waiting to see the TV commercial 1-800- BAD-DRUG. "Did you or someone you love, use opioids? One call... that's all...

As a matter of fact, I used them, 1 loved them, and I still have dreams about them. How do you reimburse me on that deal?

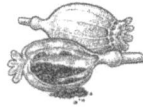

CHAPTER FIFTEEN

I now realize looking back, that my life had been driven by one big glaring factor, it was ruled by fear. It seems that most all of the decisions I made in life going forward were motivated by my reaction to this dark and gloomy emotion called fear. Fear seems to have been at the center of the nucleus that surrounded itself with a protective shield of sorts. This shield contained a number of reactive behaviors that I used to battle the life I dreaded facing every living day. The choices I made in my life, given my outlook of what lied ahead were nothing less than a bundle of decisions that bordered on self-destruction. I didn't feel that a quick suicide would be fair, such as jumping to my death, a gunshot to the head, or a quick overdose. For I was not worthy of such a quick out. No, I needed to suffer for sins as I remember Jesus had to suffer. And from the stories I remembered, Jesus was actually an innocent victim, who was defiled by the wicked people on earth. So why would I, this not so innocent junkie, not need to pay with vast punishment and suffering.

However, as the selfish human being I was, I began to find a pleasurable way of self-destruction. And it seemed that this physical feeling of euphoria lent itself to a narcissistic personality within me. Everything became about me, and how I felt. All I knew back then was that I somehow, someway, absolutely needed to drown out the guilt of my sin. And the pleasure I found in opiates became my refuge.

It always seems to amaze me that I went from feeling that I needed to suffer, to a sanctimonious outlook on what I deserved. I had gradually, though it seemed suddenly, had come to realize that I put myself in the position of going from a transgressor to a victim.

Did I ever mention the time I thought that I may possibly be too selfish and self-centered a person? Then I realized that people just didn't understand how important I really was.

It's strange how my head works when I delve into that dark corner of my mind. It seems that it has a protective mechanism that directs me in a way as to ease any emotional pain that surfaces. With that said, it's pretty much needless to say why I did the things I was to do, growing into adulthood. And rather than why, what, was the horrendous path I made and the wreckage I left behind on my journey.

Now I had to believe that I could find a way to rid myself of my insane way of life and impaired thinking. The sad thing was that I didn't even really know that I was messed up. I just assumed that life had been unfair and I fell victim to some bad breaks. I didn't even see that I was messed up from my insane thought process throughout life. I was just a victim.

One of the hardest lessons in life is letting go. Whether it's guilt, anger, love, loss, or betrayal. Change is so freaking hard. We seem to fight to hold on, yet we fight to let go. It's like trying to push two magnets together, which is nearly impossible.

A few quotes that I find ring so very true in my life, are the following;

- "I can neither love nor be loved if I allow my secrets to get in the way.

- It's the side of myself that I refuse to look at which rules me.

- I must be willing to look at the dark side in order to heal my mind and heart

- Because that is the road to freedom."

The bottom line is "Life is too short to wake up with regrets. So love the people who treat you right and forget about the ones who constantly cause strife. And, for those who bring no positivity to your life? Walk away!

What I find very amazing about my life, and so many people that I've come across through my travels here on this Earth, is the imbalance between good vs bad. It seems that within our minds, hearts, and our souls, there lies so much good, though no doubt we all have some bad. However, it is the bad, which may just be a secret, whether a deep dark secret, or just a seemingly little one, it nevertheless take center stage to all. It is almost mind blowing that even the smallest secret or negativity that people like myself have in their mind seems to be the ruling part, or driving force, if you will. It seems as though a person may have vastly more goodness in their mind, heart, and soul prevalent, however it seems to be the very smallest part of negativity or dark secrets that seem to rule the thoughts. It's almost the way of a guilt driven life, and it is always unsettling none the less. I guess I could best describe it as a beautiful pure white garment, though the tiniest of any stain will distort its beauty.

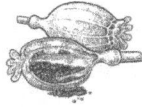

CHAPTER SIXTEEN

In early 1985, fortunately for me, I was locked up for the last time, which probably saved me from myself. It was that cold sobering day which set off the elimination of drugs and alcohol from my life.

I vividly remember that for a long period of time it was like losing the very best friend I'd ever had throughout my entire life. I had valued my relationship with heroin as if it were the god of a thousand dreams, with each dream cherished as the most euphoric state of being, which life could ever possibly offer. It was each and every bit the most magical dream a human being could ever imagine. I found that it was a dream of promise that offered a magical escape, which at the time freed me from ever feeling alone in the world. But at the end of those wonderful and fulfilling dreams that I previously referred to, comes the most horrific nightmares that can haunt you the rest of your days on this earth.

Back then I couldn't exactly figure out if I was mentally ill, a drug addict, or if it was normal. The latter sure didn't seem to ring true because when I looked around at other people, it was very rare that I noticed anyone else that lived like I had.

Even after I cleaned up and got sober, I viewed the world as one of cold desolation, with the never ending fear of deceit lurking around every corner. And it is what I lived, in my view, which was what all mankind was about, a big bowl of endless deception.

There I was, this messed up, dysfunctional man with the delusional notion that by stopping drugs and the life of crime, everything would be fine and dandy. Dandy my ass. My life had now felt worse than I had ever imagined one's life could get. If I had known then, when I made the decision to quit drugs and alcohol that my life would still be so completely unmanageable, I think I would have just taken the leap into the world beyond. Or, for whatever you may believe, whether it's just a dirt nap, a trip into an eternal fire of burning hell, or just slipping into nothingness.

Back then I felt there was no possible way to rid my mind of the seemingly endless black hole of guilt, regret, pain, despair, and endless agony. It was one big fucking nightmare. And that horrible dream reminded me during every waking moment and it followed me to my pillow each night, with whispers of hopelessness.

It's not necessarily the insane world we live in, which was and always will be a bizarre place. It's actually the stinking thinking in my head that makes the world crazy, and that's where perception is reality. And for me, whenever I catch myself in the crazy mode, I know I need to do some very deep soul searching. Or, better yet, get myself to a twelve step meeting.

One thing I do know and have witnessed firsthand about opium and all of its derivatives, they do in fact destroy lives, once you're hooked. My own experience in this arena has shown me that once a person endures opiate addiction, the proverbial seed is there to stay. This stuff somehow, somewhere, engraves a notch in both the mind and soul. It seems that once it has infected a person, that seed will manifest itself permanently. It may lie dormant for weeks, months, or even years, but it does not ever seem to go away. It is for that very reason I have found it to be imperative to eradicate it the only way I know how, which is through a twelve step program. It's a twenty four hour, daily work in progress for me.

That seed of addiction in me seems to manifest and nourish itself by way of stinking thinking. It seems to thrive on the negativity within your head. And all the while it reminds you that there is only one way to resolve the calm in the mind and soul within you. It's almost like that of plant germination, once it's fed, it will grow. And the growth of the seed of addiction is a very difficult and taxing thing to fend off.

One thing I find as a red flag for me, is when I become more and more guarded. I become overly paranoid that other people are not trustworthy. That's when I want to grab the proverbial steering wheel and turn things around. I would make a guess that people who have a difficult time trusting others probably came from a place where they likely didn't trust themselves. Or, a person who may very well have themselves been deceitful throughout life. In my case I will say that both scenarios may just fit.

Something I heard years ago, stuck with me: "Just as a snake sheds its skin, we must shed our past over and over again." I myself seem to go through periods where I make time to reflect on what in my life is working and what is not. The funny thing is I have this habit of cleaning and organizing while my mind works at figuring out what needs to change in my behaviors, and what needs to be released from life. It's always good to start new with a clean house.

And when I reflect back on a time in my life when I remember feeling periods of happiness and contentment, I try to recall how I ultimately lost it. It's then that I'd most likely know where not to look for it.

Truth be told, the admission of being powerless over my addiction was not an extremely difficult thing to acknowledge, given the war torn body, and the afflicted emotional state of hopelessness I found myself in. The difficult part of conceding was having to face the past, whereas I had lived the life of being an extremely selfish "son of a bitch", the prior thirty years.

What I found to be so very difficult in my new life of 'sobriety' was the fact that after the many years of heavy opioid use, I would eventually need to face the wreckage of my past. The reality of truly getting sober was and is, that the arduous task of repairing the damage of my years of abuse. Or, I knew I would never, ever, be able to move forward in life.

I believe I used opiates for many years to numb the horrible feelings of guilt, regret, and hopelessness I carried from about age six to age seventeen. Much of my ill faded memories were due to a dark and haunting childhood experience, where-as I felt responsible for causing the death of my, would be, youngest sister.

$$* * * * *$$

When I finally eliminated drugs and alcohol from my life, it was as if I had then regressed back to my teen years. I felt like, ok here we go, all the same old shit is here back on my lap. And now I had to deal with the likes of growing up all over again, along with all of stuff I did, while I was using opioids. So here I sat back at step one...correction...step one, plus MINUS 5.

All in all, given the history book of my life I would guess one would assess my prior life as probably not only a junkie, but perhaps a man with a very self-centered, self-serving, shell of a man, with a very pessimistic attitude, or simply put, a complete asshole.

With that being said, I at least had somewhere to start with some thorough soul searching. It would be then, and only then, that I'd be able to begin on the path to real sobriety.

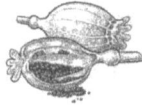

CHAPTER SEVENTEEN

While I now go into my thirty second year of being clean and sober, my thought process has changed my views on many different things.

One view I use to have' which has changed is the fact of who the real victim or victims really are in this world of opioid addiction. In my individual case I would contend that through rigorous honesty and thorough soul searching, I've come to the realization that I may have just been the victim of myself. And as the victim, I took prisoners through my ill-advised lifestyle, thus I engendered victims of my own doing. My victims were first and foremost my family, friends, and other loved ones. For that the only atonement I can make, and the only way of restoration of these relationships is by living the righteous way of life. In many cases even that is not enough to heal the wounds of yesteryear. However, sobriety is what I have to offer with the hope that it may one day be enough to bring resolve to the damages others endured, due to my insane lifestyle.

Another category of victims that my insane lifestyle affected, in a very pathetic way, were the many physicians I wronged. It was in my selfish pursuit of opioids, that I not only interrupted the care and needs of the genuinely sick, but I also contributed in causing mistrust in some physicians. And by that I may have ultimately affected the needs of the truly sick patients after me.

Truth be told, it's people like myself, while living the disgusting lifestyle I had, that have played a part of damaging the actual need of opioids for the righteously pain inflicted patients.

Unfortunately many of us make some very poor decisions. So, what I am implying is that I believe the vast majority of physicians are not at fault for addiction in patients. I am not saying there are not some bad apples in the medical field. However I strongly believe that the vast majority of doctors are good and caring people. Like I said there are a few unscrupulous doctors. In the height of my addiction I came across a few of them.

There was one that you could walk in the office and sit in line with literally 20 to 30 people in the waiting room. The well-known drill was that you'd eventually be taken to a patient room, and while waiting for the doctor to walk in, you'd have a $20 bill in your hand. You would want to be sure he could see the cash, without literally handing it to him. You would then mention that you're back hurt, mention the drug that worked best for your pain (which in my case was Percodan). The first words out of this guy's mouth were "are you going to pay me?"

Now his initial method of operation was that he'd take your money, slide it in his pocket, and he'd begin writing the prescription. It was generally a script for 60 Percodan that he'd begin writing for. But, it was common knowledge that you'd have to say something like, "I'm going to be going out of town, so could you make it 120 pills?" He would look over at you, directly in the face, and his eyes would drop to your pocket, as to look for more cash. The smart thing was to have your hand in your pocket as you requested the uptick. Hell, it was worth another $10 or $20, seeing that we were paying $3 for a single pill, from a neighbor woman. This woman was ironically in his office either before or after you. Her saving grace was that she didn't use drugs, but liked money just the same.

Now there was another doctor that we use to make monthly visits to for Dilaudid. I would go in with none other than my bad back, and request Dilaudid. It was like pulling teeth with this guy. I'd be lucky to walk out with a script for twelve 4mg Dilaudid. And the bill was in excess of $50 with this guy.

However, this same doc, different patient, 90 to 120 freakin Dilaudid. The catch was that the other patient was my buddy's girlfriend, and she was needless to say, a very attractive and shapely young lady. And she had no qualms about dancing for the prescriptions, if you understand what I'm implying. I re-member that we'd have to take her to the appointment at about 6 or 7 o'clock in the evening, and sit in the car smoking ciga-rettes waiting. Shit, some nights we waited two to three hours and go through a pack of cigarettes waiting. Then she'd finally come out throw the prescription on the dash board, and say "I fucked his brains out, so I get half." Well, she had a point, but we sat in the car for almost three hours some evenings waiting for her. I guess this doctor didn't know the meaning of a quick piece.

So yes, there are a few doctors that probably fall in the category of bad apples, as in any other profession. And the two I mentioned both just happened to fall prey to their own demons. One of which apparently had a strong thirst of greed, and the other an unusual sexual hunger.

I would be remiss if I didn't mention the truly wonderful and caring physicians I've encountered throughout my last thirty one plus years of being sober. There are quite a few physicians that I would say stand out and above any others I've encountered. But, overall I must say that visiting with a physician when you're not drug seeking is quite a different experience. That shark like attitude is gone when you're seeking care for actual pain and discomfort.

In my sober travels of the healthcare arena I can clearly see the gun shy reactions of medical professionals, when I would mention pain of some sort. I immediately get this feeling that some type of invisible shield goes up. And I don't think I'm just imagining it. I guess I wasn't the only drug seeker out there.

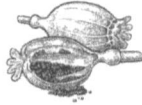

CHAPTER EIGHTEEN

What I see in the world of opioids and the making of an addict is this; it is as I've mentioned previously, its choices. I promise you that the vast number of people who are and have been addicted to opioids, are people that chose to use recreationally. I will agree that in no way did these people have the faintest idea that it would take them as deep as it probably had. I don't think anyone could even imagine the depth of the grasp that opioids can have. It digs its way so far into every fiber of a person's physical being, that it seems to take a hold of the mind and soul, through the nerves. It's that cunning and baffling.

In my many years of trying to figure out the whole opioid dilemma that we have before us in this world, it always seems that it comes back to the same old conclusion. And it's one of amazement.

Going all the way back in time to when opium was introduced into the medical profession during the 1800's, it has baffled the brightest of professionals. It sounds as though they found it to be the "cure all" for pain and many other healthcare epidemics, initially. Even to this very day it has proven itself to be deemed "the hand of God", but in that other hand it yields an evil beast.

The good that opioids have tendered to the medical profession definitely outweigh the bad. However, it is again, ultimately dependent on the choice of how and when opioids are administered.

If the medical professional truly wants to curb opioid addiction, there are definite steps that need to change in treating painful ailments. Take a patient with back pain for example. When a patient initially present themselves with enough pain that prompts a visit to a medical facility, it's obviously beyond their individual, acceptable pain tolerance.

I know everyone has their own pain tolerance, and it is what it is, as far as their acceptance, or they wouldn't even be there. The initial visit is obviously to determine the root cause of the pain, and treating the discomfort. If and when the source of the pain is pinpointed, there is no doubt a course of action that is recommended. If it's bad muscle pain, there is a reason for the muscles to react. If it's a pulled muscle due to a sudden strenuous occurrence, and either X-rays or an MRI do not show an affected nerve, it's muscle relaxer time. If the X-ray or MRI show an afflicted disc or joint, it's possibly time to administer an opioid, depending on the severity of the initial pain. What I myself have observed is lack of expediency in addressing the root cause of pain due to afflicted discs in the spine. It seems that it would be logical to administer a nerve block initially, while determining a course of action to repair the affected disc.

An example is that the patient will have the pain addressed with opioids, masking the root cause, and giving a false sense of repair of the ailment. If it's a surgical procedure that's needed to repair the cause of the nerve affliction, I say it's the only way to approach it. I've seen so many people treated with extended opioid therapy and their belief seems to be that it is cured, or that there is no cure other than opioid pain treatment. The successful outcomes that I've seen in many cases are patients where the root cause of the pain is treated with expediency. The shorter a patient is on opioids the better.

The overwhelming evidence of opioid dependency and abuse, points to the "at risk" persons. And from what I've seen, it is clearly the case that the opioid dependent person is one that pursued the drug, and not the one that the physician created. This, I believe, is the biggest miss on the part of the Joint Commission and other government agencies tracking such data.

Are there cases where a patient with no history of abuse becomes physically dependent on opioid medication after extended use? Absolutely. However, I am quite sure that this particular type of patient is also one that can be successfully weaned off opioids, and they go right back to the normal lifestyle they once enjoyed. And that, in my opinion, is the difference between the innocent victims of opioid addiction and the seekers.

I'm also quite sure that the drug seeker didn't originally set out with the knowledge that they'd fall victim to the extent that they would. But, it is an ugly fact that from outside looking in, you can clearly see that the seekers choice will ultimately result in the agony of defeat that I promise.

There is also evidence that patients who have abused legal opioid prescriptions had in prior years of their lives, used other forms of chemical relaxation methods. Whether it was marijuana, alcohol, or other drugs, it most times sends up a red flag as to strong vulnerability. I've spoken to various people during my research of patients who have had extended periods of opioid usage, due to injuries or genetic ailments.

One gentleman was a 68 year old who had sustained a back injury due to lifting. The injury had caused pinched nerves in his lower lumbar, due to the over exertion, along with common degenerative discs, which were also present in his case. The pinched nerves caused severe muscle spasms which he felt were unbearable to the point of extreme pain, while performing his regular daily functions.

This patient was given OxyContin for pain, and a brief administration of oral steroids to help alleviate the inflammation around the discs. The physician's treatment was aimed at treating the initial pain and to remove the inflammation around the disc causing the nerve from an obstructed flow. It seems to be a very common and sensible approach.

This patient's history is one of a man who never did any more than experimentation with marijuana and his alcohol use was what would be considered very moderate, i.e. A weekly glass of wine or two. He made mention that the pain pills helped with the discomfort, but made him drowsy. He made no mention of the medication being euphoric, and was not familiar with the class of drug being an opioid, or the addiction potential. His physician only made mention that the pain medication was only a short term treatment until the spinal inflammation subsided.

Six months after the initial injury, the physician ordered another MRI to observe the progress from his original state that the oral steroids and rest had yielded.

The physician's opinion was that the disc was now less obstructed, however the patient's pain still existed, though lessened. This physician then opted for a procedure using Botox, which he suggested would be an attempt to avoid spinal surgery, leaving that as a last resort. The patient agreed, and was injected with Botox into the afflicted muscles as to freeze them, so to speak. The patient was then prescribed the lessor non opioid pain reliever, Toradol, and a muscle relaxer.

After 90 days, this patient had seen significant progress, and has reported to be pain free in the area previously afflicted.

I need to say that given a very similar injury and comparable treatment for another patient I followed, resulted in a very different outcome. This patient was a 52 year old female who suffered a similar injury to the same lumbar area of the back.

The pain reported by this patient was also described as severe, with muscle spasms, which she stated had altered her regular daily work and home regimen.

One of the differing factors in the history of this patient, was her admission of periodic marijuana use, and above the norm alcohol usage, compared to the prior patient mentioned.

In this patient, who was treated by a different physician, OxyContin was also prescribed for a period of approximately six months, along with a brief period of oral steroids. This patient reported little progress in the pain levels, along with the need for more pain medication.

Now I'm neither a rocket scientist, nor did I stay at a holiday inn, but I can tell you that the progression, or lack thereof, in the 52 year old patient, would flash a caution sign in my mind.

* * * * *

It's a given that after an injury or other ailment, which a person sustains causing them pain and discomfort, commonly prompts them to seek treatment. But, there are many people, such as myself, that have the propensity to go from a pain free status, to wanting just a bit more. We want to feel better. And there's nothing like good old opioids which will accommodate just that.

For me, opioids didn't only render physical pain relief, but they eliminated the existence of mental anguish and gave me a social confidence second to none. To me, opium has proven to be exactly as it was initially described over a century ago, when it was likened to the "hand of God".

The comforting powers of opium come as a Godsend, so it seems, unfortunately it also carries with it, deep below the surface, an evil beast, so it seems. You like it? Take more...and more...and then it's got you exactly where the medical professionals warned you it would. The problem is that it's so cunning and baffling to the point of instilling complete denial when it invades your mind and soul. "What do they know" the beast will ask you, assuring you that all will be ok. And why wouldn't you believe what it tells you, it's proven to be everything you ever dreamed a drug could be, and it's never let you down. You probably never felt so good in your entire life, prior to using opioids.

The bottom line is, history has proven opium to be a savior of sorts, in relieving pain and discomfort, with nothing on earth coming even close. And there is crystal clear evidence that after centuries of vast human research and development in the way of treating pain without opiates, we've come up empty handed even to this day.

History tells us that opium and its derivatives have been and will always be the benchmark of treating pain. It's just as much a fact of life in the medical field, as it is to treating infections with antibiotics. All repeated attempts of creating that painkiller without the physically addictive characteristics have fallen short.

The fact is that opioids are here to stay is just that, a fact, and rightfully so. It has been proven to be the king of kings in the pain killing arena.

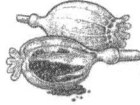

CHAPTER NINETEEN

And now as we find opioids as much a part of medicine as antibiotics, there are medical professionals who attempt to remove it as an option, except in terminal patients. In theory this seems to be a very logical and responsible approach to pain treatment. However, the cat is out of the bag, so to speak, as to a more informed public realize pain can be killed. I would guess the majority of people would opt to have a pain killer, rather than a pain reliever. And with not knowing the true horrors that addiction brings, it seems to make sense that the unknowing patient opts for opiates to be the drug of choice.

From my vast experience throughout the years with opioid usage, I encountered many different people who had opiates of some kind for sale. Between me and the circle of acquaintances I had during my drug years, it's just what we did. We made it our business to know who had cancer, who suffered broken bones, and who was going to a dentist. We knew they either had opiates or they were definitely candidates, for us to offer our professional opinions on how to obtain a prescription. But, truth be told, most times they already had some Percodan or Dilaudid in their possession.

There were seemingly spots in every neighborhood that had somebody who was selling opiates. It was anyone from a college student to some old grandmother who I bought from through the years. For some people it's the way they subsidize their finances. They know the demand is always there, so whether they need opiates for pain or for money, they do their best to keep a steady flow of prescriptions whenever they can.

My point in bringing attention to this is, the bottom line will show that people make choices. And those choices make for addicts. I would again guess, and even bet, that physicians are not what makes people dependent on opioids 90% of the time. Opioid dependency is most times inclusive of unfortunate injuries, unsettled lives, and bad choices. Many may disagree with my analogy of addiction, but I'm sorry to say that it is just what the hell it is. Choices most times due to the almighty illusion that fear instills in all of us. Once you begin to feel the wrath of physical withdrawals from opioids, it's all but over. That seed is already planted in your soul.

When an addict truly makes the decision to quit, they will intuitively know by the sign that comes from their gut. It's when their courage kills the scared little boy within himself and decides to be a man. Or, when the wisdom decides to slay the whimpering young girl within, and is determined to become a woman. It is when your gut sends that signal to the intuitive part of your soul. It tells you that the white flag of surrender has been raised, signaling a time of needed regeneration from the war inside your body, mind, and soul. And that it has all but destroyed the child within to the point of transcending to virtual adulthood. It's the transition from pain to escapism and to forbearance, which is called acceptance.

A woman once told me that her acceptance of addiction had been like that of postpartum psychosis. She said it was like delving into the unknown with nothing other than hope. It was the hope of finding refuge from a war within herself that she likened to being at the end of a cliff. And it was if she intuitively knew she would land safely, though it was that seed of her addiction, that cast doubt in her mind.

Many women will tell you that there is no pain that can reach the height of childbirth. Though the aftermath of labor brings with it an almost welcoming numbness given the pain which had been endured.

Maybe that's why men find it harder to reach the plane of acceptance? Or, maybe it's just that the proverbial cliff is closer for men? Either way, we all seem to get to the point of facing the fact that the cliff of any addict is inevitable. Though some people will leap to their death from this ugly thing called addiction.

The ugly fact for many is that after escaping the wrath of addiction, it still leaves an inflicted body with the pain which was present from the onset of their injury. And what makes it even more difficult to endure, is the fact that some of the original pain which may still exist, many times feels amplified, tenfold, due to the elimination of painkillers. It's almost as if It then says "I hurt, kill me" referring to the pain, and gives a signal to the brain reminding you how well the opioids worked.

What makes pain so unbearable in the person who has been tainted by opioid dependency is the seed which made its way to germination inside the afflicted mind. It takes center stage and begins to dictate what needs to be done to correctly relieve the pain, your body is telling you it has. It seemingly amplifies the known true pain a person has, and says "kill it without prejudice"!

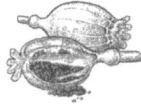

CHAPTER TWENTY

In January of 1977, I was inpatient at a hospital for drug treatment and I kept hearing the word "fear" in our group therapy sessions. In my free time, I continued to think about it and continued to look at the word. And in this crazy head of mine I kept trying to decipher it. I found myself writing the word and while deep in thought I found it to be "false evidence appearing real".

When you think about it, the reality of the word is that it's one of the most prominent factors that many times prevented me from moving forward in life's pursuits. On the other hand it's an intuitive quality that can keep us alive. That's what makes fear such a cunning and baffling property of life.

On one hand you have to respect fear and on the other you want to destroy it, and all that it represents.

What is so interesting about fear is that it can preserve life and on the other hand prevent life. What other word can be described so adversely different in the aspects of how it can alter a person's life.

The way I live my life today is the only way I know how, one day at a time.

Twelve step programs seem to clear a path in the brain amidst all of the stinking thinking and seemingly jumbled up chaos that resides in this head of mine, most of the time. It's almost as if it clears a path in your mind to logic. Without logic being the prominent part of your brain doing the work, you are all but lost. And you're then making decisions based on emotions instead of self-preservation.

What I always find so intriguing is the fact that when I began my trek into the world of being clean and sober, is that I wanted no part of it. The cold truth is that I had exhausted every bit of energy I had, both physically and mentally. It was even after Endocarditis, broken syringe needles floating in my extremities, Hepatitis C, extensive circulatory problems, and cellulitis, I still wasn't done. Since my heart was still beating I felt I could stand a bit more self-torture and destruction.

However, there was one factor that prevented me from continuing on the path I was so intent on completing. It was the legal system that had intruded its way into my life's path.

I had also exhausted my behind the scene "ace in the hole", or secret advantages, if you will. Not even a friendly and sympathetic judge I had close by could justify letting me continue my personal rampage of sorts. I had become a danger to myself in every way imaginable, and my fate was sure death.

My story is only one of millions that have gone through the fury of opioid addiction. Mine was one of abuse, whereas many people that were, or still are struggling with it were in fact mere victims of opioid addiction by just wanting to be pain free.

Nevertheless, when it has you in its grip it doesn't care how you became dependent, it sends the same monkey to visit all of us. That monkey is there to remind you just how good you felt at the most pain free and peaceful moment it gave you during the worst of times. It all just seems so unfair that it works so damn well, but like a thief in the night it steals a part of you, which feels as if you'll never be normal again.

With all things said, there definitely is hope. One of the biggest issues surrounding opioid addiction is the fear that it instils in the dependent person. It's a mechanism that seems to be built into the makeup of opioid effects on the mind. Once it has proven itself that it will eliminate physical pain, and it will, it has already infiltrated the persons mind. Once it's in your mind, it will do its best to convince you that it is to be trusted. And it's then when a person is comfortable enough to allow it to become your crutch. It not only becomes a crutch in making you confident that it is the one and only real option for physical pain, but your emotional fears are also eliminated by its effects. It also gives a sense of confidence to the addict whereas without it, you'll feel completely lost. It thrives on being the all in one source of total being, delving deep into the soul. That's no doubt where the old saying, "selling your soul" came from. And believe me, you would if you could, for just one more fix.

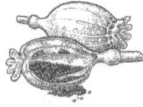

CHAPTER TWENTY ONE

There have recently been a number of revolutionary discoveries, in the realm of pain. One in particular surrounds the element of the memory, in its correlation of addiction, which looks to be very promising.

There is a gentleman by the name of Todd Sacktor that through some astonishing research found something called PKMzeta, which is the "engine of memory". It's something that is definitely way over my head, though in reading the results that were recorded in Todd Sacktor's discovery, it shows that there is hope in erasing the memory of pain.

He apparently carried out an experiment with rats, where they zapped the cells with electric pulses to create strong connections between them. Then they injected a chemical called ZIP, which blocks PKMzeta. After the injection, he discovered, the long-term potentiation disappeared. Todd Sacktor became convinced that PKMzeta wasn't just an important molecule. He decided it was necessary and sufficient, on its own, to lock in memories.

It basically says that it is the memory of pain stored in the spine. It's an amazing discovery that could possibly change the world of pain as we know it.

The whole concept of bringing something like this to fruition would be an absolutely groundbreaking find that could drastically change the way of pain management.

However, as with anything else in the realm of science, there just may be other ramifications that come about from it. There are the skeptics that question how it may affect other parts of the memory. The possible benefits from a concept such as this, were it successful, would be voluminous.

Maybe when God created me, it was just a bad day for installing PKM zeta. For me physical pain is not pleasant, probably like most other people, however I find emotional pain much more excruciating. I am definitely not the most pleasant person to be around while suffering emotional pain. That is where I firmly believe opioids affected my emotional wellbeing. I used opiates so much, and for so long, that it seemed to numb much of the normal growing pains in life that my emotional nerves had gone haywire, and seem to have become extra sensitive. I have been physically beaten more than a few times throughout my life, in as far as auto accidents, and other various mishaps. Make no mistake about it, I'm not implying that physical pain is a pleasant experience. What I mean to say is that emotional pain for me, is a horrific feeling, and I'd take a physical beating over an emotional beating, any day.

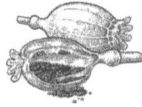

CHAPTER TWENTY TWO

Another interesting theory that I have found to be fascinating, which I myself cannot dispute, is that a defective dopaminergic (neurons which release dopamine) within the human brain could possibly exhibit the difference between a true "addictive personality" (my opinion of the definition of the "At Risk" patient) and the "normal" functioning person.

There is much evidence pointing to the fact that people with "Dopamine deficiency" are extremely prone to having addictive personalities. It's pretty much a given that if a person has the deficiency present, it points to various symptoms present in the persons makeup, such as low energy, demotivation, and even suicidal tendencies.

Opioids flood the brain within the dopamine receptors, thus awakening the "happy neurotransmitters" in a person. With people who already have a "dopamine deficiency", in my opinion, are seemingly immediately enamored when opioids hit the brain. It not only relieves or kills the pain, but it seems that the dopamine receptors spike up dramatically, as opposed to persons with normal functioning dopamine levels.

When administering opioids to a person with normal functioning dopamine receptors, it would appear that they do in fact relieve or kill the pain for which they're prescribed, however, I've noticed they state a sleepy feeling. The sleepy or almost dream state of which opiates produce, do seem to mirror the physical feeling likewise in persons with, and without dopamine deficiencies. However, it seems that the person with a deficiency not only achieve pain relief, but also appear to entice their dopamine levels to highs they just did not have prior to administering opioids.

For me, there is no such thing as moderation, planning, or rational thinking.

There's definitely something to the dopamine deficiency theory that hits home with me as to what seems to differentiate someone like me, no doubt the deficient type person, from the normal person. I truly believe that it is where you will see the difference between dependency and addiction.

I imagine anyone would become dependent over an extended period of time being treated with opioids. The withdrawal of opiates definitely has an actual course of regeneration within the neurotransmitters and physical familiarity the drugs had been supplying, and occupied itself within the patient. It's the person with the prior dopamine deficiency that is not only subject to the regeneration of the healing process within the body during withdrawal, but it also seemingly hijacks the dopamine producing function it enjoyed while using opioids. Now that is almost like that person in the desert finding the cooler full of ice and water, only to be a mirage.

Along with the normal, or common, physical withdrawals the dopamine deficient person experiences, it is also the seemingly abrupt theft of their dopamine producing source, that finds this person completely distraught and debilitated, sometimes to the point of becoming deeply depressed, irrational, and even suicidal. It's as if their entire life, over time of extended opioid dependency, it had become the one and only dopamine supplier they came to know and depend on.

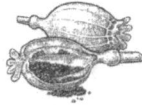

CHAPTER TWENTY THREE

For many years now, I've watched closely the coverage of opioid addiction in our society. I've also periodically read up on the progress, or lack thereof, in respect to the various government agencies involved with the healthcare system.

For one, the FDA (Food and Drug Administration) which seems to continually approve various different opioid drugs. There's one with a binder which is to help prevent it from being easily injectable. Another adds another binder, to inhibit nasal inhalation.

All while approving more new concoctions, it seems they find the need to have a regional or nationwide seminar for the agencies to discuss warnings. I'm sure there is a need for good communication as to educating healthcare professionals, however, my research has found that they are very costly. And from what material seems to come out of them, it's almost ridiculous.

Educational progress coming from the FDA and similar agencies have failed dismally over the past 30 plus years. The communication to the public should be very clear cut, forthright, and precise in the warnings. When I consistently see new warning labels every 6 months, whereas one or two words have changed, I wonder how much this has added to the average taxpayer's bottom line.

What is very obvious is that these warning labels have done NOTHING.

The educational information that I would hope to see is exactly what I described earlier, in that inevitable ramifications of extended opioid use are certain. They are promised to be difficult. This is not a category of drugs like marijuana, amphetamines, or some others that "could" be addictive. Opioids "are" physically addictive in long term use.

In 2016 the FDA spent over 1 Billion dollars on targeting opioid use, abuse, and warnings. In my research I found that nearly all of the budgeted expenditures went toward meetings, which came up with these results: warning labels upon warning labels for prescription opioids.

If anyone really believes that these "warning labels" have done anything to curb opioid abuse, they are sorely mistaken, it's a joke. I always wondered how much it actually cost to add the "Do not operate heavy machinery" label on opioid prescriptions.

The FDA is no doubt wonderful at keeping food safety at the top of its game. But when it comes to the particular subject of opioid safety, they seem all but completely lost and oblivious to reality. It's the FDA that approves opioid drug products as frequent as the weather changes in the Midwest. It seems to be a new concoction with opioids being the main ingredient, every month. And the further I looked into the approval process they take, I get more confused. And, what tells you that it's dysfunctional is that there are new class action lawsuits against drug companies being announced weekly. The FDA almost appears to be feeding lawyers by approving a drug, and a short time after, the drug is deemed a danger to patients. The ones held accountable are the drug companies, and ultimately seems to find patients blaming those damned doctors. And, who ultimately ends up paying for everything mentioned above? We the people.

There is a legal concept known as "sovereign immunity" whereas you cannot sue the FDA for approving a drug that is later proven to be defective and dangerous. What a concept that is.

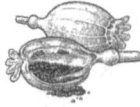

CHAPTER TWENTY FOUR

It was in the late 1990's that the Veterans Administration began using pain as the "Fifth Vital Sign". And in 2001 the "Joint Commission" picked up the concept and thus began "Pain" the Fifth Vital Sign".

For those of us (a guy like me) that have heard the term "Vital signs" but really never completely understood what they actually were, is best described as the following;

Vital signs are measurements of the body's most basic functions. The four main vital signs routinely monitored by medical professionals and health care providers include the following:

1. Body temperature
2. Pulse rate
3. Respiration rate (rate of breathing)
4. Blood pressure (Blood pressure is not actually considered a vital sign, but is often measured along with the vital signs.)

Vital signs are useful in detecting or monitoring medical problems. Vital signs can be measured in a medical setting, at home, at the site of a medical emergency, or elsewhere.

The whole idea of the concept was brought about due to an attempt to find some way to gauge pain. Caring for the sick and afflicted most always finds that a patient is displaying pain in some way or another. Whether its pain or discomfort, it's important just the same. So, the idea of pain being a "vital sign "does make sense in a way that would warrant it as it is almost always present. An example would be what I envision, is if you could look into a person's retina and get an actual gauge of just how much pain was present. To me, that is where pain could actually warrant a reason to deem it as a "vital sign".

And, as we also know there is pain, and there's discomfort. Both pain and discomfort are the body's way of indicating something isn't right. I would imagine that it's not very common that a guy wakes up one day and says, "Honey, I'm feeling pretty damn good today, I think I'll just take a quick ride to an urgent care and pick up some morphine tabs."

Now the whole idea behind making "pain" a "vital sign" was to somehow find a way of accurately treating pain by prescribing pain medicine accordingly. And opioids have obviously been the drug of choice for any medical professional treating "pain". And it is for good reason that opioids have almost always been the go to drug. You can't beat opioids in treating physical pain, you just can't.

There's a reason drug companies have used opioids as the platform in which to emulate, and they have actually been trying this for over a century, to no avail.

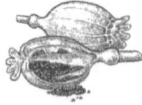

CHAPTER TWENTY FIVE

Below is documentation I found about the details on Pain, the "fifth vital sign". I'm not a medical professional, in fact I barely made it through high school. But I will be chiming in with my comments just the same. The reason I do, is that after viewing the following articles, I see that egos and pride affect even the most highly educated people. Possibly more so than other not so educated people, such as myself.

I wrote my comments and opinions in bold italics.

Statement on pain management from David W. Baker, MD, MPH, FACP, Executive Vice President, Healthcare Quality Evaluation, The Joint Commission:

In the environment of today's prescription opioid epidemic, everyone is looking for someone to blame. Often, The Joint Commission's pain standards take that blame.

MY OPINION / COMMENTS:

This claim is riddled with hypocrisy. It states they're taking the blame. Really?? Look at the following statements, and tell me they aren't actually pushing the blame.

We are encouraging our critics to look at our exact standards, along with the historical context of our standards, to fully understand what our accredited organizations are required to do with regard to pain.

The Joint Commission first established standards for pain assessment and treatment in 2001 in response to the national outcry about the widespread problem of under-treatment of pain. The Joint Commission's current standards require that organizations establish policies regarding pain assessment and treatment and conduct educational efforts to ensure compliance. The standards DO NOT require the use of drugs to manage a patient's pain; and when a drug is appropriate, the standards do not specify which drug should be prescribed.

Our foundational standards are quite simple. *(Simple??)* They are:

- The hospital educates all licensed independent practitioners on assessing and managing pain.
- The hospital respects the patient's right to pain management.
- The hospital assesses and manages the patient's pain.
- Requirements for what should be addressed in organizations' policies include:
- The hospital conducts a comprehensive pain assessment

that is consistent with its scope of care, treatment, and services and the patient's condition.

MY COMMENT/OPINION:

(It's my understanding doctors always have assessed pain, and treatment was done accordingly. It's something they learned in medical school.)

However, it should also be noted only a few employees of the Joint Commission actually went to medical school.

This seems extremely hypocritical in the respect that physicians always had assessed pain and always have taken in to account their patients wellbeing. It's what they've always done.

And most hospital organizations manage their physician's treatment of patients, by way of review boards headed by actual medical professionals.

The hospital uses methods to assess pain that are consistent with the patient's age, condition, and ability to understand.

MY COMMENT/OPINION:

(I heard that this too was taught in the first year of medical school, is it not?)

The hospital reassesses and responds to the patient's pain, based on its reassessment criteria.

MY COMMENT/OPINION:

(Ok, let's add another step to the process? Stupidity. It adds more busy paperwork and required documentation while other patients wait to be seen. Now, how much does this add to healthcare costs, as well as hamper the care of patients waiting to be seen. Not to mention that it could ultimately be the difference between life and death for a patient, waiting while the required documentation is being logged.)

The hospital either treats the patient's pain or refers the patient for treatment. Note: Treatment strategies for pain may include pharmacologic and nonpharmacological approaches. Strategies should reflect a patient-centered approach and consider the patient's current presentation, the health care providers' clinical judgment, and the risks and benefits associated with the strategies, including potential risk of dependency, addiction, and abuse.

MY COMMENT/OPINION:

(The Joint Commission seems to be saying that doctors need to treat pain how the patient's see well. And then go on to say; "ok, now don't make them addicts, people.")

Furthermore, physicians are continually educated on new strategies of pain care treatment by actual medical boards, compromised of experienced physicians, not lay people given a manual of does and dints in medicine.

Despite the stability and simplicity of our standards, misconceptions persist, and I would like to take this opportunity to address the most common ones:

MY COMMENT/OPINION:
(Simplicity?? WTF? This has the smell of a government agency trying to justify their existence.)

Misconceptions would have never existed, had our government stayed out of this aspect of healthcare.

Misconception #1:
The Joint Commission endorses pain as a vital sign

The Joint Commission does not endorse pain as a vital sign, and this is not part of our standards. Starting in 1990, pain experts started calling for pain to be "made visible." Some organizations implemented programs to try to achieve this by making pain a vital sign. The original 2001 Joint Commission standards did not state that pain needed to be treated like a vital sign.

MY COMMENT/OPINION:
(Note that it states doctors and nurses do not have to treat pain like a vital sign, however they just better have all of the pain assessments logged in the patient records, or they risk the possibility of not being reimbursed for the care given.)

If it is, as the Joint Commission claims, not a vital sign, why then is it that in recording patient assessments, treatment, and discharge notes, where reimbursement is sometimes denied.

Then it is where physicians are required to give detailed follow up information, explaining the reasons it may not have been addressed. And, this no doubt takes additional administrative time away from physicians, and ultimately takes away from actual face time with current and waiting patients.

It sounds very time consuming and unnecessary.

The only time that The Joint Commission standards referenced the fifth vital sign was when The Joint Commission provided examples of what some organizations were doing to assess patient pain. In 2002, The Joint Commission addressed the problems in the use of the 5th vital sign concept by describing the unintended consequences of this approach to pain management and described how organizations had subsequently modified their processes.

Misconception #2:
The Joint Commission requires pain assessment for all patients.

The original pain standards stated "Pain is assessed in all patients." This was applicable to all accreditation programs (i.e., Hospital, Nursing Care Center, Behavioral Health Care, etc.). This requirement was eliminated in 2009 from all programs except Behavioral Health Care Accreditation. Patients in behavioral health care settings were thought to be less able to bring up the fact that they were in pain and, therefore, required a more aggressive approach. The current Behavioral Health Care Accreditation standard says, "The organization screens all patients for physical pain."

MY COMMENT/OPINION:

As far as Behavioral Health patients are concerned, using a more aggressive approach? I do understand that the "aggressive approach" may not insinuate being verbally aggressive with the patient. And, to imply that a more in depth look at the patients underlying symptoms which may be causing pain, is understandable. But, that's just what the mentally ill don't need, is for a physician to use a more aggressive approach.

Maybe you tell them they're lying and they need pain meds? With the mentally ill, they're already in pain in their mind, so probing them more may not be the answer.

The majority of mentally ill patients downplay pain. So, the only real option is to let them know you care about how they're feeling. This too, is merely a common sense approach.

Misconception #2 (*continued*)

the current version of the standard for hospitals and programs other than Behavioral Health says "The hospital assesses and manages the patient's pain."

This standard allows organizations to set their own policies regarding which patients should have pain assessed based on the population served and the services delivered. Joint Commission surveyors determine whether such policies have been established, and whether there is evidence that the organization's own policies are followed. Some organizations may still follow the old standard and require pain assessment of all patients.

MY COMMENT/OPINION:

The Commission says it allows hospitals to assess pain by the individual hospital standards. However, they just better meet the Commission standards, or again risk denial of payment for services rendered. That is a clearly documented fact.

Misconception #3:
The Joint Commission requires that pain be treated until the pain score reaches zero.

MY COMMENT/OPINION:

Ok, in misconception #1 it states JC does NOT endorse pain as a "vital sign". And here in #3 it states the JC does not require that pain be treated "until the level reaches "0" Zero as in the "vital sign" scale of 1 to 10.

If you're not endorsing the scale, why then would it ever have been a misconception?

The JC doesn't mention the fact that if a patient's pain levels, or care, haven't been clearly addressed and logged in the records, reimbursement of services may just be denied. Am I missing something?

Misconception #3 (continued) there are several variations of this misconception, including that The Joint Commission requires that patients are treated by an algorithm according to their pain score. In fact, throughout our history we have advocated for an individualized patient-centric approach that does not require zero pain. The introduction to the "Care of Patients Functional Chapter" in 2001 started by saying that the goal of care is "to provide individualized care in settings responsive to specific patient needs."

MY COMMENT/OPINION:

Providing individualized care to specific patient needs has been the standard since the inception of medical care by physicians.

Furthermore, providing care to the specific needs of the patient, as physicians have done throughout the history of medicine, points to the fact the JC utilizes patient complaints, as to what the patient feels they need, or want.

It's as if to say that a patient will determine whether or not their needs were met, thus determining reimbursements to hospitals and physicians.

Misconception #4:

The Joint Commission standards push doctors to prescribe opioids. As stated above, the current standards do not push clinicians to prescribe opioids. We do not mention opioids at all:

MY COMMENT/OPINION:

The Joint Commission may be a bit misinformed. The fact is that nothing works as well as opioids for real pain. As physicians are told to be careful and use opioids only as a last resort, that's a good thing. But, the fact remains that when a patient leaves the hospital and the so called non opioid pain meds fail, patients complain. And when patients complain, the Commission asks why doctors are not properly treating pain. It's a double edged sword. Let doctors listen to patients as they do, and let doctors treat patients the best they know how.

Most hospital organizations already monitor doctors on their care based on patient comments and complaints, by way of medical professionals reviewing each individual physician's care of their patients.

Misconception #4 (*continued*)

the note to the standard says: Treatment strategies for pain may include pharmacologic and nonpharmacological approaches. Strategies should reflect a patient-centered approach and consider the patient's current presentation, the health care providers' clinical judgment, and the risks and benefits associated with the strategies, including potential risk of dependency, addiction, and abuse.

MY COMMENT/OPINION:

Now when the hell did doctors NOT use their best judgement to treat their patients?

Misconception #5:

The Joint Commission pain standards caused a sharp rise in opioid prescriptions.

This claim is completely contradicted by data from the National Institute on Drug Abuse. The graph below (Figure 1 in the report) shows the number of opioid prescriptions filled at commercial pharmacies in the United States from 1991 to 2013 shows the rate had been steadily increasing for 10 years prior to the standards' release in 2001. It is likely that the increase in opioid prescriptions began in response to the growing concerns in the U.S. about under treatment of pain and efforts by pain management experts to allay physicians' concerns about using opioids for non-malignant pain. Moreover, the standards do not appear to have accelerated the trend in opioid prescribing. If there was an uptick in the rate of increase in opioid use, it appears to have occurred around 1997-1998, two years prior to release of the standards.

The Joint Commission pain standards were designed to address a serious, intractable problem in patient care that affected millions of people, including inadequate pain control for both acute and chronic conditions. The standards were designed to be part of the solution. We believe that our standards, when read thoroughly and correctly interpreted, continue to encourage organizations to establish education programs, training, policies, and procedures that improve the assessment and treatment of pain without promoting the unnecessary or inappropriate use of opioids.

The Joint Commission is committed to working to dispel these misunderstandings and welcomes dialogue with the dedicated individuals who are caring for patients in our accredited organizations.

MY COMMENT/OPINION:

This entire statement from the Joint Commission has the smell of an attempt to rid themselves from blame. It is completely contrary to their opening statement of this article.

Then the "Commission" seems to come up with some graph defending their existence and pushing the blame on physicians, which once again furthers their case in justifying their existence. Bizarre.

Furthermore, I heard that a representative of the "Joint Commission" supposedly made a comment pushing the bulk of the blame in the spike of opioid use and abuse toward emergency room physicians overprescribing. I've got news for the Joint Commission. The majority of overprescribing and use of pain meds were occurring prior to most patient's initial visits to the emergency room.

Mark my words that if a historical study is done in the realm of patient visits to emergency rooms, you will undoubtedly find the use of opioids were already present in the patient records prior to the initial visit. And in many cases, history will no doubt show patient use of street drugs i.e. Heroin, OxyContin, etc. prior to the visits.

Another fact the "Joint Commission" fails to mention in this statement of misconceptions, is the fact that they endorsed opioid prescribing in 1996, backing "Purdue Pharma" claims that opioid condemnation was way overblown.

This thing, opium, and its byproducts, are bigger than anything in the history of addiction, mankind has seen.

What's sad is the constant blame game, which is nothing but a big bowl of out of control professionals diverting the fact that they're just not as bright as they would contend. Blame takes people out of the accountability department, thus brushing the real issues under the proverbial rug. And, it's the oldest "hot potato" scenario that runs throughout most every big business organization.

They take a problem that seems hopeless in solving, pass the buck, and blame the doctors. It's a smart move, because there are a lot of physicians and the "Commission" knows the "hot potato" will land on someone's lap, other than theirs. And it does seemingly bounce around and never, ever, lands. And all the while the public says "those damn doctors, look what they've done now". Pay no attention to that "Commission" behind the curtain. Nothing to see here folks. And of course, it once again furthers the case of their very existence.

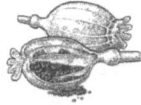

CHAPTER TWENTY SIX

(Below is an article from a separate "Pain Report")

The nation's largest medical society is recommending that pain be removed as a "fifth vital sign" in professional medical standards – a move critics say will make it even more difficult for pain sufferers to have their pain properly diagnosed and treated.

Delegates at the annual meeting of the American Medical Association in Chicago also passed several other resolutions aimed at reducing opioid prescribing and increasing access to addiction treatment. The AMA represents over 200,000 physicians in the U.S. and is very influential in setting public health policy.

The AMA's new president said physicians played a key role in starting the so-called opioid epidemic by overprescribing pain medication, and now must do their part to end it.

"We have taken ownership of that, and physicians have taken ownership of being part of the solution," AMA president Andrew Gurman, MD, told Modern Healthcare.

The AMA's main "solution" to the opioid problem is to stop asking patients about their pain.

MY COMMENT/OPINION:

It seems logical that if someone is going to a doctor he's probably suffering from discomfort of some kind. And if they're in pain, they're probably going to mention it anyway.

It sounds very much like Dr. Andrew Gurman, M.D. gets it. His statement is a very noble and humble way of accepting the physicians, whom he represents, possible mistakes. It appears he is taking accountability for mistakes made on behalf of AMA members, which may have played a part of the current opioid epidemic before us.

Pain was first recognized as the fifth vital sign in the 1990's, giving pain equal status with blood pressure, heart rate, respiratory rate and temperature as vital signs. The policy encourages healthcare providers to ask patients about their pain.

But critics say pain is not a vital sign, but more of a symptom, and cannot be measured like a patient's temperature or blood pressure. They also claim the "Joint Commission" a non-profit agency that accredits hospitals and other U.S. healthcare organizations, sets pain management standards too high, which contributes to opioid overprescribing.

MY COMMENT/OPINION:

The above statement makes perfect sense. Whoever wrote this hit the nail on the head? It is the Joint Commission that has waffled on pain management policies. And I would contend the Joint Commission seems to have historically made decisions based on emotions.

First off, let me just say that every person on this earth has different pain tolerance and varying slide scales. It's absolutely absurd to even think that a 1-10 sliding scale can be used in pain management. Plain stupid I say

"Just as we now know (the) earth is not flat, we know that pain is not a vital sign. Let's remove that from the lexicon," James Milam, MD, an AMA delegate said in MedPage Today. "Whatever it's going to take to no longer include pain as a vital sign ... Let's just get rid of the whole concept and try to move on."

MY COMMENT/OPINION:

Well stated Dr. Milan, MD, Throw that concept in the trash, and mark it up as a valuable lesson learned, as not to put the person who came up with it on the defensive, prolonging the needless battle of furthering the 'blame game'. .

"I am astounded that physicians don't believe we should assess pain on a regular and ongoing basis. That is exactly what removing pain as a vital sign means," said Lynn Webster, MD, past president of the American Academy of Pain Medicine and vice president of scientific affairs at PRA Health Sciences.

Webster says dropping pain as a vital sign would setback pain care three decades.

"The problem is that too many physicians and policymakers equate assessing pain with giving opioids," he said in an email to Pain News Network. "It appears that advocates for removing pain as a 5th vital sign are suggesting that if we just ignore pain then we won't have to deal with pain and opioid abuse will disappear. That is not only fantastical thinking, it is harmful to millions of people in pain."

MY COMMENT/OPINION:

Dear Dr. Lynn Webster, MD, going back three decades may not be a bad idea. There were less opioid scripts written and less opioid dependency / addicts. Back then they'd rub dirt on it.

Let me ask you this doc, If I give my hangnail pain a 10, what would you suggest I get, 120 OxyContin?

Sarcasm aside, I do agree pain should not necessarily be equated to what opioid to prescribe, and what dose. There are many different sources of pain, and various options for treatment.

However, as I've mentioned earlier, a pain scale is not a bad thing, though it is something that just cannot be gauged with anything other than perception.

And I disagree that it is somehow harmful to anyone at all. The real problem with it as a vital sign is again because it subjective and speculative.

For example; Back spasms could be described as a '5' whereas I would imagine would be treated with muscle relaxers and anti-inflammatory. Contrarily, kidney stones at '5' would most likely be opioid time.

Below is another professional's opinion;

"This is a very unfortunate decision, (eliminating pain as the 5th Vital sign) one that creates the very real possibility that we will see a decrement in the quality of pain care delivered in various institutions," warned Bob Twillman, PhD, Executive Director of the Academy of Integrative Pain Management.

"The Joint Commission standards say you need to assess pain in every patient; record the results of that assessment; provide some kind of treatment; re-assess to see if the treatment was effective; and teach staff how to manage pain. They do not say we should ask patients how much pain they have on a 0-10 scale and give them opioids until the pain level is 4 or less. Not asking about pain does not make pain go away, and it does not relieve healthcare providers of their moral and ethical obligation to treat that pain effectively."

MY COMMENT/OPINION:

After reading the prior statement, all I can say is; I now believe I have a very good idea on why healthcare costs are rising.

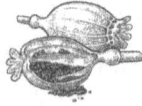

CHAPTER TWENTY SEVEN

The bottom line is that opioids are here to stay, and rightfully so. The shit is that good, believe me.

So, as for terminally ill patients with pain, leave them the hell alone. What are you worried about, addiction? They're on their way out, leave it alone. Let them choose it as if they were going into a candy store, and allow them as much as they want.

I barely have a high school education, though I honestly believe I could be more useful in the way of proposing solutions, then some of the book smart medical professionals. But, the whole idea of the "fifth vital sign" is ludicrous because it adds unnecessary steps for physicians and medical staffs which is a time consuming waste of valuable time and money.

Here they come up with this sliding scale of 1-10, with smiley faces down to sad faces? Now tell me, who the hell is honestly supposed to determine pain levels by this concept? Whether I'm a junkie, who's always marking a 10 with a crying face, or an innocent old grandmother who is in severe pain, but too proud to even select a 5?

My mother, a World War Two army nurse, would no doubt say, "oh, there are people worse off than me" until she gets home, and you can see she's obviously in terrible pain. She lived her life in a time that the "Great Depression" hit, and hurt. People were just grateful they had food. If they were hurt physically they were told to rub some dirt on it. Ok, I know that was almost one hundred years ago, and we don't need to live with pain, given the medical advances since then. My point is that I say again, pain has and always will be subjective.

I remember a time when I was about 12 years old, I hurt my leg playing football. I went home and asked my mother what I could do about the pain. She simply said, "Rest it for bit. There are some people who don't even have legs. You don't know what pain is."

Well, I still have the freakin leg, mom. All I wanted to know is if there was any way to ease the pain.

In her defense, having been an army nurse, she served in the Philippine Islands, and treated young boys who lost their limbs, and many who lost their lives.

Knowing this, I realized that the subjectivity of pain is so very much one of perception, which varies from person to person.

I guess the idea of deeming pain the fifth vital sign was well intentioned, but it's stupid just the same. Don't get me wrong, asking a patient what level they'd rank their pain at, from 1 to 10, with 10 being unbearable, is understandable. However, what I find ridiculous is, that with pain as a vital sign apparently requires physicians and nurses to log an entire new line item recording it in the patient records.

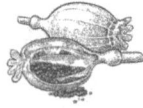

CHAPTER TWENTY EIGHT

As I've mentioned numerous times, the cold hard fact is that opioids are hands down the most effective on most any pain.

And it's also a fact that when a patient walks out of a clinic or hospital and the Tramadol they're given does nothing for the pain but make them sick, there's a quick complaint filed.

This is where "Press Ganey" comes into the picture. "Press Ganey" is a company that was founded in 1985, which claims to support healthcare providers, by assisting them in understanding and improving the patient experience.

In my research of "Press Ganey", I am of the opinion that they too deserve a large portion of the blame for our skyrocketing opioid epidemic.

"Press Ganey" not only monetized their concept by selling the surveys they produce, but in turn, they also offer consulting services, by claiming to enhance patient satisfaction. Patient satisfaction is a good thing, make no mistake about it. But, what I found to be so very interesting, is the fact that this organization, in its travels throughout the healthcare industry, has become, in most cases, "THE" determining factor on how hospitals and its physicians are graded, and ultimately affects the monetary reimbursement to the hospitals and physicians. And, keep in mind that patient satisfaction doesn't necessarily mean quality patient care. It may be a good gauge of how the patient felt about how they were treated, however, I believe most all of us would have to agree that this in reality has little if nothing to do with the quality of the outcome for what they were treated for.

If I were to write a review for how I was treated, it could very well be based on how I felt that given day. I may not like how the doctor smelled that day, and answer the survey grading him below average for being a smelly son of a bitch, that did a superb job in correcting my physical ailment.

So, the problem I've seen with this entire process, is that the "Joint Commission" has more or less, in my view, used the "Press Ganey" reports with their conclusions of the patient satisfaction surveys, and has ultimately become a benchmark in determining reimbursements to hospitals and physicians.

In other words, my view is that the "Joint Commission" is holding the hospitals and physicians by the balls, and telling them if they refuse to play nice, reminding doctors whose sandbox they're in.

My question is, how did this organization become to be so influential to the point of directly affecting the monetary outcome of healthcare services?

Am I wrong in contending that physicians have been getting screwed every time they turn around, in the way that they have been shown a new hoop to jump through, seemingly at the drop of a hat?

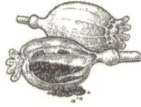

CHAPTER TWENTY NINE

I do not profess to know, or expect that even a keenly trained physician knows with any amount of certainty when pain described by a patient is real, or not. So, that is I believe, where the complaints submitted to hospitals and organizations like the "Joint Commission" via "Press Ganey" have hit a home run, so to speak, for the addict types, like myself. It has become a weapon for drug seekers to pull out that "can of whipass" the "Joint Commission" supplied us with, in their confrontation of physicians who were being stingy with the power of their pen, in writing scripts for opioids, and we knew it.

When I hear the Joint Commission's view that it is the negligence of physicians being the main driver of creating addicts, I say with extreme confidence, in making my assertion, that it is absolute BULL SHIT.

I say the vast majority of doctors are not the problem. With all due respect, I must say that I completely disagree with the Joint Commissions contention.

Furthermore, I would remind the 'Joint Commission' of the old saying, *'People in glass houses should not cast stones'*

Can you blame a tavern or bartender for creating an alcoholic? No.

Now I understand that may be like comparing apples to oranges in the way that a person ordering a drink is knowingly making a choice that is their own personal business. But, I will tell you this, guys like me can twist the situation of requesting opioids from a physician, in the same way, with the same argument of sorts.

Yes, if that patron of the bar finds that he is an alcoholic, it's on himself. And, when a patient requests an opioid prescription, the physician can deny such treatment, and send the patient to a pain clinic. Now, I will never deny that there are vast differences between someone ordering a drink at a bar and requesting opioids from a doctor. However, I do believe that the recent assertions and actions of the "Joint Commission" have in fact closed the gap between these two paradigms, whether or not they want to admit it.

Yes, I'm quite sure that the scenarios I've described will be used as a very ludicrous example. But, I tell you that it has become so very true, in my opinion, when comparing the two, due to the "Joint Commission's" prior contentions and reactions.

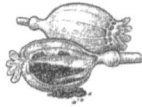

CHAPTER THIRTY

Again, I must say that the recent insinuations made by a number of "Joint Commission" staff employees, stating that emergency physicians play a large part in creating the recent abuse of opioids, due to their liberal opioid prescribing practices, to unknowing and innocent patients they've treated, is a crock of shit. An average opioid prescription given by emergency medical professionals is 12 tablets.

The fact is that after the initial ER visit, which the said injury or painful condition that the patient was originally treated for is referred for follow up with their primary physician, or specialist. And it's then, that a patient can then easily point out that they have already been prescribed opioids. And, the "at risk" type, I guarantee, will state that the opioid is the only thing that worked for their pain. There definitely are very authentic and honest to goodness ailments and injuries that in fact do warrant opioids, as they do work wonders with pain. I guarantee it.

I will tell you this, it is that the truly innocent patient seeking pain relief for their condition in their follow up with the specialist or family doctor, the vast majority of times, won't even bring up the subject of which type of pills they need. They just trust the judgement of their physician to treat it as they see fit. That is just a fact.

Another fact is that if the patient being seen for follow up specifically mentions the opioid pain pills they were prescribed, with insistence they need more, it is there you have an opioid hunter, I promise you.

I believe that the use of "Press Ganey" reports, which are gauged by patient reviews, is where the distortion of the facts, and the broad sense of physician abuses, paints a very different reality, as opposed to what is probably in actuality a story that is factually somewhere in between the patients perception of their care, and the physician's diagnosis and treatment. But, for "Press Ganey" to report patient complaints as the gospel, is where the real problem lies. And, it also lends way for animosity within physician / patient relationships and interactions.

I say this as my opinion, due to the "patient bill of rights" reference, in which the "Joint Commission" pointed to, inferring that there may possibly be sanctions for inadequate control of pain.

I don't contend that there should not be a "patient bill of rights", however, I do not believe that using it in reference to dictating how physicians should and should not treat pain, is wrong. One fact is that I'm quite sure it's the patients right to choose another physician, if they do in fact feel the care is inappropriate.

But, using the patient bill of rights as a tool in threatening physicians with sanctions, is in my opinion, a typical government approach to using sanctions as a tool to control physicians, by way of threat. The patient bill of rights should be to eliminate government from interfering with the actual patient's choice of treatment.

It's a fact that many physicians felt coerced by the "Joint Commission" into being more liberal with opioids, and some ten years later, appear to be blamed for overprescribing. Does this not sound like the typical government style bull shit in play here?

I know that it is not an easy task in grasping the whole opioid abuse trail. It is in fact, a very cunning and baffling case of insanity that began with a tiny little poppy seed, which grew to become such peace in ridding pain. And, it has definitely proven to be a Godsend remedy, especially in treating excruciating pain incurred by terminally ill patients with cancer. This is where the "hand of God" description fits so very well when defining what opium's purpose could very well be.

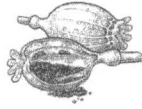

CHAPTER THIRTY ONE

Here's my view on how this whole mess with our healthcare system began, how it has evolved, what it is now, and the correlation with the opioid epidemic.

First of all, physicians, for the most part, are not business savvy people by nature. There's a reason they went into medicine, and most physicians will tell you the business side of it, is the biggest pet peeve of their practices.

That is where we had the influx of businessmen gaining control of hospitals and ultimately their physicians, by way of shrewd business practices. Then it is where medicine progressed to a very competitive landscape, which catapulted to promotion and marketing. Thus we began to call it "our healthcare system"

Then organizations, such as "HMO's" backed by politicians edged their way into the medical field by way of assertion that more laws and regulations were needed in healthcare. Their contention was that they wanted to protect and uphold patient rights.

The current trend in the healthcare industry, and I say industry, because big business minds saw an opportunity to cash in on healthcare, as a shark sees blood. Yes, there was some need to put a taste of business sense into the medical field due to the growing knowledge of cures and treatments. But these guys just seemed to have bullied their way in taking over healthcare, thus deeming it the healthcare "industry".

You have to admit that it was a smart move on their part. They've penetrated the hospitals with their relationships with drug companies, hospital equipment businesses, and hell, they even penetrated our government and legal professions.

It also sure seems to have given everyone involved, lucrative payouts, on a healthcare industry that's losing money at an alarming rate, partially due to the very existence of big businesses involvement in the industry.

What other business do you see with billions of dollars in bonuses coming out of a losing business?

And now what do we have? Politicians and business people pointing their fingers at physicians, suggesting they are overpaid, and a big reason for escalating medical costs. Forget the fact that physicians owe educational tuition for years. And pay no attention to the questionable business practices that are part of the makeup in today's healthcare industry.

Now we see another influx of government entities wedging their way into healthcare to get a piece of the pie. Again, I agree there needs to be some rules and regulations. But the reason for this, is the fact that our healthcare system was made an industry in the first place.

At the very inception of organizations, like the "Joint Commission", there probably were some very well intentioned aims of supporting physicians, while supporting patients also. Unfortunately, organizations such as the "Joint Commission" gradually became a branch of our government, and went from a support system, to a controlling system, and ultimately began forcing its will on hospitals and the physicians.

And thus, we see costs of healthcare slowly, but very surely, rising to astronomical proportions.

But, of course it's for the good of the people.

Now consider the current climate in which insurance companies are threatening refusal of payment for inappropriately treated medical conditions.

In the case of pain management, which is a subjective patient experience, the quandary of medicating vs not medicating, can bring with it, the price tag of differentiating between the births of dependency vs a patient left to suffer.

It's a smart move on the part of the Joint Commission and insurance companies, whereas they cover all their bases. Unfortunately for the physicians, they find that they're damned if they do, and damned if they don't. And the outcome for the patient many times ends up in suffering due to the medical professional being apprehensive in their approach toward treating pain, with the ultimate goal of being compassionate and empathetic toward the patient care.

I guess you could say that the bottom line is that when you have business people making decisions for medical care, you find a disconnect that most times results in chaos. And this is where the medical profession now finds itself.

And now, we the people, find ourselves in the hands and care of our government. Yes, it is another big business empire which has delved its claws into what is best for our mental and physical health. The hypocrisy is that they won't touch the very healthcare coverage that they tailored just for us. "It's going to be great, just wait and see. Yeah? You try it first. Then show me this wonderful, special plan you specifically tailored just for us. Better yet, take your snake oil and after your mother uses it, then talk to me.

My point is that the cruel fact of addiction is complex enough without having the government or insurance companies intervene. Funding is one thing, and yes, some regulation is probably necessary, but a government agency run by business people dictating physician care has proven to be a nightmare. Just look at these clowns writing nearly 20,000 pages of regulation for our dictated healthcare. What a sad joke it is. And now I ask you, do we really want these agencies mandating physicians on what pain meds we need?

The problem has come from the overbearing control of the government roll in medicine, which it has virtually snatched away from physicians, and the rest of the medical professionals. It has also seemed to force its will on physicians in the way of dictating how to practice, by way of more government agencies structuring how hospitals need to perform. And the performance measures, are ones they came up with. They will tell you that they have intended this whole structuring process is to put healthcare back in the hands of the people.

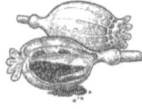

CHAPTER THIRTY TWO

So, now as I myself sit and read some of the regulation attempts of opioid dispensing, I do have to laugh. I do not laugh at the fact that this stuff has proven to destroy lives, tear apart families, and probably cost taxpayers more than anything else in our country. The reason I laugh is because if you look at all of the money and resources spent to corral the use and abuse, i.e. Healthcare costs, law enforcement, prisons, hospitals, insurance costs, and on and on. And we now dare have our government become more involved in fixing it. It's actually the government that has had a major role in screwing it up in the first place.

I've worked at some larger corporations, and I've seen firsthand, the layers of departments and positions that exist in many big companies. And I become nauseated thinking back on how difficult it was to get things done. It's actually just plain disgusting when I think back on it.

There were many times people in the position of power, making decisions based on a few customer complaints, without hearing both sides of a story. And, these same people in the positions of power, were most times people who they themselves, never held a position that dealt directly with customers.

And it appears we've now succeeded in building our healthcare system on the same platform of sorts. The alarming thing here is that we're talking about people's lives, in this scenario. But no, we need to create layers of positions, upon positions, of employees gathering unsubstantiated data, that are almost certainly useless and skewed facts that are presented as the gospel. UN fucking believable. Drain that damned swamp, before it's too late!

If we would just get these clueless clowns in Washington out of the healthcare business, let doctors be doctors, and let us, the people, decide on our own, by way of our educated choice, in choosing our fate with the trusted healthcare provider of our choice.

There is just too much wrong with the way things are controlled in this new order of government and business people running healthcare.

There is evidence that much of the influx of opioid abuse can be linked back to the 2001 Joint Commission pain standards being set, due to the public outcry on the undertreatment of pain.

It was then that we saw the "Joint Commission" come down on physicians for not properly treating pain. Thus we are where we are on the new addict blame game. I'm telling you, this opium shit is by far the most cunning and baffling dilemma in medicine, and has been for some time.

Well, as the good old boy network in America will always operate, we then saw things like deals being made for buying hospital supplies from a guy, who knows a guy. And then of course, we have the instances that has reared its head in healthcare for many years, where drug companies infiltrate the hospital systems with their new go to meds.

And then we may have seen one of the biggest shams of the 20th century, and up through the present time, in the world of medicine. The Purdue Pharma marketing subterfuge.

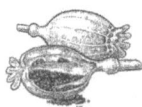

CHAPTER THIRTY THREE

In 1995 Purdue Pharma came out with the drug "OxyContin". And, in their marketing promotion they featured statements by well-known physicians, most prominently, Dr. Russell Portenoy, who is renowned as a health care leader, in the medical world. Dr. Portenoy is Past President of the American Academy of Hospice and Palliative Medicine and Past President of the American Pain Society. He previously chaired the American Board of Hospice and Palliative Medicine, and Chief Medical Officer of MJHS (Metropolitan Jewish Health System) Hospice and Palliative Care at Mount Sinai Beth Israel Medical Center.

Dr. Portenoy stated in promotional materials, which "Purdue Pharma" the maker of OxyContin produced in their marketing campaign, he said that opioid addiction was way overblown.

Dr. Portenoy stated that there was a "total lack of evidence" regarding long term opioid usage in chronic and non-cancer pain management, causing dependency. The promotion also made mention that less than 1% of patients using the drug became addicted, and overdoses were extremely rare. WTF?

Though I believe Dr. Portenoy's glorification of opioid treatment of pain is probably sincere, and also on target of the fact that opioids are a "Godsend" in treating pain. As I've mentioned so very many times, there just is nothing on this earth that even comes close, in comparison.

However, when he states that the risk of opioid addiction when prescribed by a doctor, is extremely low? And less than 1% became addicted? How criminal!

Keep in mind the fact that this man is a very highly educated physician, with many years of experience in the field of hospice care, which most likely points to extensive opioid familiarity. Along with the glaring fact that he has practiced in New York? In my opinion, he sounds very much like the guy in the story who came out of the shelter after a tornado, saying "ain't it grand the wind stop blowing", seemingly oblivious to the wreckage that lay strewn across the land. Well, in this case, some ten years after hitting the market, the wreckage is a voluminous number of fatalities due to OxyContin overdoses.

For a physician with the credentials Dr. Portenoy has no doubt earned throughout his professional career, seems to have stuck his head in the sand, if he truly believes the statement he proclaimed in his promotional material stating "the likelihood of patients treated with opioids for pain will lead to addiction is extremely low, when prescribed by a physician."

Another interesting fact is that Dr. Portenoy taught about pain management, while practicing in New York.

All the while, the nearby morgues were probably filled with

opioid overdose victims, hospitals filled with cases related to opioid abuse, the prisons overcrowded, with many of the inmates incarcerated due to drug related crimes, and the streets flooded with so many lost souls affected by opioid abuse.

Now, if you want people to accept the fact that you truly believe your own opinion that the risk of opioid dependency is extremely low? Shame on you, Dr. Portenoy.

Over 16,000 people die each year from opioid overdoses, and as many as 30,000 in the past year, you money grubbing prick.

I guess when you're financially entangled with the drug company promoting one of the most potent opioid concoctions produced to this day, you may tend to be a bit biased. My personal opinion is that the statement he made, when used in the promotion of an opioid, is as criminal as it could possibly be.

On the part of "Purdue Pharma" using this well-known physician in the promotional materials, it was an absolutely brilliant move. I could see how physicians throughout the medical field just knowing the credentials of Dr. Portenoy, and hearing his message in the promotional piece, would be almost be viewed as the gospel.

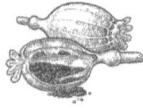

CHAPTER THIRTY FOUR

In May 2007, Purdue Pharma pleaded guilty to misleading the public about OxyContin's risk of addiction, and agreed to pay $600 million in one of the largest pharmaceutical settlements in U.S. history. Its president, top lawyer, and former chief medical officer pleaded guilty as individuals to misbranding charges, a criminal violation, and agreed to pay a total of $34.5 million in fines. The executives are: Michael Friedman, the company's president, who agreed to pay $19 million in fines; Howard R. Udell, its top lawyer, who agreed to pay $8 million; and Dr. Paul D. Goldenheim, its former medical director, who agreed to pay $7.5 million.

In addition, the three top executives were charged with a felony and sentenced to 400 hours of community service in drug treatment programs.

Okay, let me ask you: in the scenario of a street level drug dealer who was selling OxyContin to someone, and while exchanging the pills for cash, warned the buyer to be extra careful when taking the pills, because people have died from overdosing on the stuff. And, subsequently the buyer overdosed and died from the pills he purchased from the said street dealer.

What do you think happens to the guy who sold him the Oxy-Contin, even though he was forthright and honest about the dangers of the OxyContin? Of course, the guy is probably going to do at the very least, ten years in a state or federal prison.

Am I implying that the street level dealer should be rewarded for the fact he was honest when selling the victim the pills? Hell no, he should still do time.

My point is, that the sentences handed down in the case of the Purdue Pharma executives, in my opinion, were a slap on the wrist to them, and a slap in the face to our society. It's the century old state of affairs in our country, whereas the good old boy network are seemingly most times, able to buy their way out of jail time.

The fines handed down were a joke, as each one of the executives go back to their lavish homes, probably driving the most expensive cars, at the end of each day. All while there are morgues being filled with the victims of OxyContin overdoses. Not to mention the many innocent physicians who fell prey to the deceitful marketing promotion presented to them. And now, these same physicians who were duped into the contention that the stuff was safe, are now toiling over the vast numbers of patients they sent home with OxyContin, knowing that it's a matter of time before they see the wrath of addiction and even deaths that came from their very pen.

In 2012 Dr. Portenoy stated in an interview, that according to the pain standards of 2012, that he may have presented misinformation. And he stated "we didn't know then, what we know now, regarding opioid addiction".

Are you kidding me, Dr. Portenoy? Would you have made that statement if you weren't in someone's pocket? I would contend that you probably would not have.

And to think that so many people in the medical profession probably heeded Dr. Portenoy's promotion of OxyContin as very credible, due to his historically upstanding credentials? Shame on you Doc! You may want to consider donating your proceeds from this despicable promotion to a charity associated with helping opioid addiction?

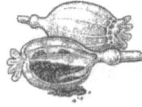

CHAPTER THIRTY FIVE

I believe that inquiring minds may want to know the whereabouts of the Joint Commission, between the 1995 and 2015 timeframe, while all of the deception by this drug company's marketing push was in full swing, destroying the lives of so many people.

This is where I found some very disturbing facts regarding the "Joint Commission" statement (outlined in CHAPTER TWENTY FIVE) of the established standards for pain assessment and treatment, published in 2001.

I was probably one of the guys crying about the reluctance of physicians to prescribe opioids prior to 1985. Maybe my voice was finally heard.

In all seriousness, back then my outcry for opioids was based on my own selfish opioid addiction.

After I read through the "Joint Commissions statement on pain", I realized that Dr. Baker neglected to mention one very important fact, when presenting his entire statement.

He forgot to mention something the Joint Commission did in 1995, which in my view, may have been one of the biggest blunders ever made in the history of medicine.

In the statement by Dr. David W. Baker M.D., while representing the "Joint Commission", whereas he addressed the 2001 standards of pain, he failed to mention a very crucial and possibly game changing fact. It was what the "Joint Commission" did in the 1995 timeframe, which in my opinion, helped jumpstart this entire opioid epidemic that we now have before us.

What you may find is that some of the following information regarding documented facts, which were verified by a report in the "Wall Street Journal", may just make you sick to your stomach. And, given the disturbing nature of how the information was conveyed, you will probably agree that it did in fact, play a big part in our current opioid epidemic, and the voluminous number of deaths, associated with it.

Well, I can't honestly tell you where the "Joint Commission was in 1995, but what I can tell you is, what they did in 1995.

They went so far as to publish a pain management guide sponsored by, none other than Purdue Pharma, on pain management WTF?

Yes, they actually published a guide which reportedly stated, "Some clinicians have inaccurate and exaggerated concerns about addiction, tolerance and risk of death. This attitude prevails despite the fact there is no evidence that addiction is a significant issue when persons are given opioids for pain control."

I am absolutely astounded that this kind of literature would be allowed to come out of an agency that runs our healthcare system. In my opinion, this was either the most deceitful thing, or the most idiotic act that has ever played out in the history of medical blunders. It is in my opinion, criminal.

Look at how many lives this epidemic has absolutely ruined. It's actually mind boggling that this would even be considered to be acceptable. Any other type of business that would make this type of error, their executives would no doubt be brought up on criminal charges.

Now, who in the hell would allow such literature to be published?

It's almost like asking the fox to publish a guide of safety measures in securing a hen house. WTF?

What did the Joint Commission expect Purdue Pharma to say in their guide on pain management, the same year they came out with OxyContin? It's extremely addictive and may even cause death? Well, obviously they did not.

Whoever gave the Joint Commission the reigns to the medical system in the first place, should be deported to the moon? Just think, we wouldn't even have to put up a wall. Un- f****ing-believable.

And the fact they turned their heads while this marketing push was going on? How many lives were ruined in the time period that they directed physicians to be more compassionate in regards to treating pain.

And, it is likely that most physicians throughout America would agree with my contention, which is that the major factor which led to the floodgates being opened, and where the OxyContin epidemic began.

Another fact is that OxyContin contains exactly the same synthetic opioid drug formula, oxycodone, which has been in painkillers, Percodan, Percocet, amongst other highly addictive opioids. And the same drug, oxycodone, which has been around since 1916, is what Purdue Pharma uses in OxyContin, except for the fact that it was a more condensed version, with no additives. Pure oxycodone!

Any person viewing the fact that OxyContin was being deemed as virtually non-addictive, should have their head examined. The mere fact that "Oxycodone" the same ingredient in Percodan, and still is in Percocet, was recognized as highly addictive as far back as 1964, when it became regulated, more closely.

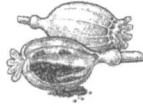

CHAPTER THIRTY SIX

Let me put the scope of the opioid epidemic into a clearer perspective.

The only way I can imagine the feeling, how many physicians may have felt when they found the whole Purdue Pharma marketing piece featuring Dr. Portenoy, was a big sham, was sometime between the ages of about 8 and 10 years old, I found the whole Santa Clause thing was a big fake. I remember feeling devastated, because I had believed in him, and I felt deceived by my gods, who were my parents, at the time.

Well, as physicians went about their practices, they seem to migrate towards the teachings of their idols and mentors in the medical field. These gods, were for many doctors, their superiors, who were their teachers and professors. And many of their said mentors, may have been envisioned as gods of sorts, based on the credentials they had earned, by way of honesty, integrity, and hard work.

Why would most physicians not trust the very hand of their mentors that fed them the knowledge and best practices of medicine that played a key role in developing them to become doctors in the first place?

And in his case of OxyContin, vast numbers of physicians took heed of the message that was portrayed by this prominent physician. A man whom had much in the way of entrusted credibility, which he had no doubt earned throughout his career. And not to mention the confidence the Joint Commission displayed, in its trust and belief of Purdue Pharma.

It wasn't until years later, after so many disturbing stories of addiction and scores of overdoses that loomed over the physician's heads, by way of having trusted this so called expert. And the very influential and trusted agencies, such as the Joint Commission, on the safety of OxyContin, which turned out to be one of the biggest frauds known to medicine.

And, it appears that the whole promotion was ultimately fueled by just plain greed, and carried out by clear cut deceptive marketing.

Now, I probably come from what some may categorize as being a 'true deplorable', given the life that I led for so many years. And, I am quite sure that this entire book will be met with attacks on my credibility, due to the scornful manner in which I've described my opinions.

However, I believe that the credentials I do possess, having been well educated in deceit, tools of greed, criminal behaviors and manipulation, along with my experience with white collar crime, have provided me some wisdoms that most living people do not possess.

With my vast people skills and a keen sense of detecting dishonesty, whether in myself or others, has shown me that it is not only drug addicts that display excessive deceit. The fact is that people infected with greed, will go to any lengths to get what they want, and the greed in this case, may just surpass the degree of plain deception, and there appears to be no cure for that.

Greed was, and still is, the one evil that ignites all of the worst, in the way of power, control, and gluttonous amounts of money. It buys things, and things are what ultimately drives greed. It's the want for having what is ultimately making lives as comfortable as they can get. It's about power, and it's about control, which is what catapulted opioids to where they are. Opioids are the ultimate comfort, and they were the key to control, in this case.

Unfortunately this is where companies such as Purdue Pharma, the maker of OxyContin, made their way into medical practices, in the way they did, by way of a brilliant marketing strategy and government influence.

In their marketing strategy, which again, was just f****in brilliant to the nth degree. They produced one of the most deceptive marketing promotions that may just be one of the all-time genius sales pitches. They used a number of physicians in their promoting OxyContin, and other opioids as being extremely safe and virtually non-addicting (quote: less than 1% addiction rate). Along with an almost nonexistent mortality rate.

The very sad fact is that one of the biggest reasons our healthcare system is so screwed up, and so damn expensive, is that big business, and our government, had jumped into the arena, thus making healthcare the expensive and dysfunctional business it has become.

And, this is where various opioids seemingly snuck their way into the picture by way of government officials being influenced by greed, power, and control.

In my opinion, it is that we were duped by our government by allowing such a sham, with the likes of the deceptively contrived marketing materials, which Purdue Pharma promoted. And to think that guys like Dr. Portenoy would stoop so low as to give the statement he did "the risk of addiction by treating pain with opioids was very low, and that overdoses were extremely rare". And, not to mention that these physicians are on record stating that opioids have very minimal addictive characteristics? Shame on those son of a bitches!

How do you think the following scenario would go over; Let's say Dr. Portenoy would happen to have an unfortunate accident, physicians have him prescribed high doses of Oxy-Contin for say, 6 months? And then have his mother wash his mouth out with Narcan? Then put him in front of the camera for a video promotion about the minimal risks of opioid dependency. I wonder how that one would go over.

I would venture to make a guess that any medical school graduate, whether it be a new resident physician, or a well-seasoned veteran of medicine, would probably agree with my opinion, and my assertion, that the statements of Dr. Portenoy, in the promotional materials, are not only very deceptive, but also outright despicable. And, I would say that despicable, is sugar-coating it. I cannot even stress enough in words how deceptive I found that statement to be.

And I would again say that if there were facts that backed the Joint Commission's statement implying that physicians have played a big part in our current opioid epidemic, it most all can be attributed to the horribly despicable, misleading messages that were conveyed by Purdue Pharma, Dr. Portenoy, and the Joint Commission. And I'd be remiss in not mentioning "Press Ganey", which in fact has just recently removed the question from their survey, regarding pain. Was this an inadvertent admission of guilt on their part, due to all of the current media given to this epidemic? Was it a desperate attempt to save face? I'd say both, in my opinion.

I would also contend that our current opioid epidemic, namely OxyContin has played a significant role in fueling the heroin uptick that has recently occurred over the past 5 years, or more.

We have a very sad state of affairs before us in this country due to the absolutely despicable, and in my opinion, criminal, conspiracy that took place.

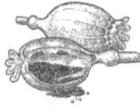

CHAPTER THIRTY SEVEN

Well, now before the medical professionals across the entire country sits that big, fat, ugly elephant in the room. They were told to be more attentive to pain, and now required to document pain to the point of possibly being denied reimbursement for their services. Almost in the same breath, they're told to stop producing addicts.

It's quite obvious the Joint Commission gave in to pressure and made a decision based on emotions. And, I think it's time to step back, forget the blame game, and regroup. There's an old saying, "Keep it simple, stupid."

I've got news for the so called professionals about the claims that doctors are producing opioid addicts. It's all a big fraud. I contend that at least 80% of the estimated "physician induced addict" numbers being thrown around are complete bull shit. And I firmly believe that 80% is an extremely high guesstimate.

If one would have an ear to the street, I'm quite sure you'd see that probably 90% of the opioids used are by choice. Granted, the disclaimer would be that you remove the terminal cancer patients and such type of persons being treated by way of supervised home care. Though I would also contend that a small percentage of those patients, opioids are either sold or stolen, for use or sale.

I would also say that after 1996, you could postulate that the other 10 to 20 percent of person's dependent on opioids, were in fact innocent and unknowing patients, who were caught up in the OxyContin subterfuge. And if you want to add to the list of victims, given this contemptible scheme that played out with all of the guilty parties, it's a large number of physicians.

I cannot sit here and tell you that I have all of the answers to eradicate opioid abuse. Nor can I give the solution as to the opioid prescribing do's and don'ts. However, what I can tell you is that the blame game and the failure of accountability definitely does not fix it either. The blame game does nothing except drive a wedge into group problem solving.

I think what needs to happen is that instead of playing the blame game, the Joint Commission needs to come up with a sliding scale for the stages of a patient's pain, in a historical level maintenance view, as to determine what category of pain management is necessary in patient care.

In this I mean, possibly a timeframe restriction for opioid prescribing in cases of outpatient care, whereas a person being treated with scheduled drug categories 1 and 2, would have a ceiling or time limit, and then move the patient to long term pain management clinics.

It's a very few people that are oblivious to the fact that opioids are addicting. And I also do not believe that doctors, with the exception of a very rare, and minuscule, group of deplorable physicians that are handing out opioids as a way to keep repeat patients.

What we now seem to be witnessing with the opioid dilemma, by way of healthcare professionals uniting to find solutions, conversely it seems to be eerily similar to the typical government gridlock we see in Washington, and it's all while patients suffer. So very sad.

When I see commissions being considered by our government to address the opioid epidemic, I feel both encouraged with the attention that it is finally being given. However, on the other hand, I cringe.

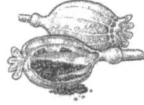

CHAPTER THIRTY EIGHT

In looking back at the year 2001, I clearly recall the aftermath of 9/11, and the encouraging signs all of Americans witnessed. It was immediately following the 9/11 disaster, that we saw both sides of our government unite in support of bringing our country together, and finally walking away from the government in-fighting.

Well, we all know how this evolved.

It actually didn't evolve, it revolved, back to the same old blame game, giving a ridiculously dysfunctional message to our entire country. What do you think the youth of our country see in the constant bickering, name calling, and verbal attacks, and destructive behavior of our so called professional adults, running our country? There is no negotiating within the government, it's an attitude of my way or the highway. It's like of bunch of people with no real life experience to speak of, making decisions for the people in real life situations. They're like a bunch of whining spoiled brats. Nice example for our school age children I'd say.

I'll be very honest, even knowing what I know now, if I were back in my teen years, and saw what our kids are seeing amongst our so called government professionals, and both sides of our media, I too would dive into drug use, head first. It's so ridiculously ugly for our children to see this country in the state that it is currently in. And now we hear people asking, "Why on earth are people doing so many drugs?"

And then we're just baffled when people coming from some impoverished and oppressed parts of the world, look around our country, and want to blow the freakin place up?

Well maybe, just maybe, it's because both sides of our media and government officials are telling Americans that either way, the end is near. Why the hell not bury our heads in a cloud of drugs to hide from what both sides are predicting?

I think we need to wake the hell up!

Do we really want our government to address solutions? I do, however I foresee another ugly blame game in the very midst of it, dashing the hope of ever getting anything resolved.

Hey, where is our drug czar, anyway?

The absolute bottom line of the epidemic we have before us, is greed and ultimately control. Both sides of our government want control. How do they get control? By votes. And how do they get votes? By painting an ugly picture of the horrible opposition party they're up against. And why? Because it benefits them.

And you ask who the big puppeteer behind all of it is? Big businesses driven by greed, which has given them control of both political parties, by supporting both sides. Every one of them want to win, because winning is everything. Winning regardless of the morality of what they may be peddling. In this case, it's the opioid epidemic. What else could give such power and control to have whatever they want, as does opium?

The solutions to opioid prescribing and addiction will never be perfect, I promise. Furthermore, the guidelines of future solutions will undoubtedly never be black and white, either. There are way too many variables in the world of pain. If there are ever going to be perfect guidelines it will only be accomplished by having a separate guideline for every person walking the earth. Opium takes no prisoners. Remember that.

As I've stated, I am not a medical professional, nor do I profess to know more about medicine, with the exception of opioids. And I'm quite sure that there probably are some guidelines being taught in medical school regarding "at risk patients" in the realm of opioid addiction. If not, it may possibly be something to consider, if it's not too politically incorrect.

What I can tell you is that an "at risk" patient in this arena is anyone whose life is chaotic in the way of being emotionally unstable, psychologically a malcontent, or just plain depressed. I strongly believe that a person with any such factor mentioned are your "at risk" patients.

Anyone with the said factors will no doubt find a refuge in opioids like no other. Any pain, discomfort, or unsettled issues a person has, will fall into dependency on these drugs. Ok, I may have just described about 90% of the patient population. But, my point is that these factors definitely play a part in opioid abuse.

In my opinion, it seems that the "Joint Commission" and other such agencies, appear to be dismissive or just possibly overlooking the fact of addiction as a disease, versus dependency, that the Commission seems to imply physicians are creating.

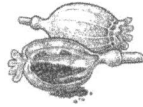

CHAPTER THIRTY NINE

In the case of a patient suffering severe pain from an illness or accident, pain thresholds may vary. A good example would be of a person who was the victim of an auto accident who endured a broken femur. During and after surgery the patient is administered opioids. Severe pain from that type of injury is no doubt present for at least six weeks. There is nothing that says ok, the six weeks are up, pain should be gone. There are so many different variations of pain tolerance from patient to patient. And, also many different healing properties that come in to play given the initial injury sustained.

What I see in these type of scenarios are the necessity of setting realistic expectations for aftercare. I'm quite sure this is a common practice that most all surgeons address when releasing a patient from a hospital stay, to home care.

What makes patient care in the realm of treating pain so arduous for a physician is that every single patient has different pain tolerance. And whether it's due to the physical makeup of the patient, or the expectation of pain the patient has, it's a huge bowl of guessing. But, I would again contend that there are factors that do point to "at risk" patient characteristics.

And what characterizes an "at risk" patient too is a very slippery slope, especially in our society given political correctness. Not to mention that it takes rigorous honesty from the patient being evaluated. I know, you're probably thinking, how the hell you are going to label someone an "at risk" patient since the whole idea of it is so complex and subjective. Well, the whole thing of addiction is complex and subjective. It's just a fact.

I went through so many different phases while attempting to eradicate the grasp opioid addiction had on me. What I found is the only thing that helped me get out of the vicious cycle of addiction was a twelve step program. I'm not implying that it's the only way, as there are many different scenarios of how the dependent person became addicted in the first place. But, if the grip of opioids keep creeping back into your life, the twelve step programs may just be the answer.

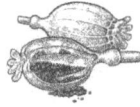

CHAPTER FORTY

Now, here we see the medical professionals and even some of the most brilliant business minds, attempting to corral this beast, to no avail.

There can be no argument that opioid abuse is a major complication in our society. It has also proven to be a huge problem, in as far as crime statistics throughout the world, not to mention vast health related issues and even deaths associated with it.

Opium is what it is, and it just can't be beat, for what it was obviously put here on earth for. I don't think anyone could dispute the fact that it works wonders, especially since there are attempts to limit its use, rather than eliminate its use in medicine, completely.

The reality of pain management has been, and always will be subjective.

Let's take a root canal. I've had a few. And a few of them were for the sole reason to get Percodan or Dilaudid, at the time. Now take a person having all four wisdom teeth extracted in one visit. Do every single one of these people need 30 tabs of Vicodin, Percodan, Dilaudid, or similar? The answer is yes and no. I had all four wisdom teeth pulled in one sitting. I had sore jaws, of course, but I did fine without opioids. Ibuprofen worked fine in my case. But, the guy next to me having the same procedure, may just be better equipped with 30 Percodan to get through it. How the hell is anyone to say its right or wrong as far as a pain scale goes? Everyone tolerates pain differently. Sure there are obviously other methods as there are different aches and pains. Ibuprofen is a wonderful drug for many basic ailments.

Take back pain. I would pull opioids, or at the least have them as a last resort. Back pain is muscle related 99% of the time, as long as cardiac issues, kidney problems, or severe neuropathy are eliminated from the equation. And for muscular problems there are many options better than opioids which only mask the pain anyway.

Some people respond well to chiropractic care and others think its voodoo.

Granted, muscle pain can be the result of many different underlying issues, however, the initial treatment can very easily, and better, be treated without opioids. There are in depth evaluations that can be done to get to the core of the problem, which are commonly spinal related afflictions. Yes, there are many other possible causes, but I can tell you this, opioids are not the answer for back spasms and such. In fact it most times will be detrimental in the way of almost certain dependency.

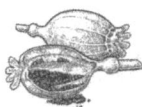

CHAPTER FORTY ONE

In the meantime, there certainly are some steps that the medical profession could take to the "Joint Commission" so to speak, in an attempt to clean this mess up.

Number one, and most importantly, if a person is in a terminal stage of cancer, eliminate with rationality, the restrictions on opioid use. Who the hell cares if they're addicted, as long as they don't mind? They're on their way out, why the hell would a doctor have to say, "I think you may be getting addicted, and there are regulations I need to follow." Leave them the hell alone. Move on to the practical interventions of the regulations by addressing the known repeat offenders. With the medical records being electronic nowadays, you should know if a patient is bouncing around from emergency room to emergency room, or pain maintenance clinic to another. And the bottom line with this is, evaluation. Is this a patient that may just be in the category of terminal or chronic, in the way of a physical disability? Is it a situation that deems they probably will have ongoing, lifelong pain? Then, you punt. You move on. They go in the pain management clinical category.

I do realize that there are risks of this particular abuse that may end up tangled in legal liability worries for physicians. But that is where some safeguards need to be put in place for the physician, possibly in the way of contractual agreements with the patient and/or their loved ones.

It seems to me that the litigation in liability lawsuits are what ultimately starts the blame game in the first place. Not to mention that this is another financial line item which came into the mix of healthcare cost spikes. Lawyers, it's a love, hate, relationship with them. There's no doubt that people need to be protected by way of having the right to litigate the possibility of malpractice in the care they receive. It's kind of like going in to have a gall bladder removed, and the doctor accidentally removes the liver. Ok, I jest. Not sure that one ever happened.

But, in reality mistakes happen, and unfortunately bad results do come out of a very small number of treatment mishaps. There are, as we all know, some not so good physicians. And even with some of the most highly regarded physicians, accidents do happen. But, this is a subject for another conversation about healthcare and malpractice reform.

Now, when the Joint Commission would get to the other stages of managing pain treatment of the dental and physical accident categories. These are generally in the short term prescribing categories. No doubt a dentist would prescribe a one-time opioid medication aftercare treatment for their patient with a root canal, as an example. Or, an emergency physician a onetime opioid prescription for broken bones, kidney stones, and such. And then it's on to the patients follow up physician. If it's then not deemed a chronic diagnosis, it's treated for a maximum six month treatment plan. From there, any and all lingering pain complaints would be referred to pain management. Then, it's on the doctor, the patient, and their family to monitor and determine whether it's chronic or terminal.

I say let the doctors practice medicine, and take them out of the babysitting role, of which goes beyond practical care, that is.

The problem, again, has come from the overbearing control of the government roll in medicine, with a plethora of deals and transactions that fly under the radar, and benefit the greed of many. And, they will again, contend that they are just there to help people and police the physicians and hospitals. They care about their constituents, of course. Maybe some of them do.

But, if they do in fact structure medicine the way they run the rest of the government, we may as well forget about it.

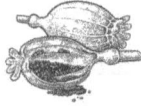

CHAPTER FORTY TWO

ow, the most important and telling question I have for everyone is, are we as a society actually committed to corralling opioid abuse? More importantly, are drug companies and our government truly willing to invest in a real solution?

Here is one safeguard that could possibly assist in curbing opioid abuse. With all of the modern day technology, here is a question that I pose as a possibility in monitoring opioid dispensing in patient care. Let's say that we have a dispenser bottle that contains 120 OxyContin tablets for a patient that is prescribed 4 tablets daily. The dispenser with a built in gps microchip could trigger an alert with each tablet being dispensed from the said patient's pill bottle. This type of dispenser is definitely achievable, and at a very reasonable cost. Though it would be a hell of a lot more expensive than your everyday pill bottle, it is a doable solution. And it may just be the cost of doing business for drug companies wanting to sell their products while offering a viable safety measure.

The alert from the dispenser could automatically be logged into the encrypted databank software, which could be viewed by the attending physicians, at their leisure. If there are signs of abusive self-dispensing, the physician could make a decision on future care or terminate the said patient.

Could the trackable tamper proof dispenser be broken into or stolen? Absolutely! But, there again you have data to back up your future opioid management for this patient.

Though this sounds insane, I truly believe it could be a very viable option in monitoring pain and curbing abuse.

Take a step back a minute and look at all of the many feeble, time consuming, expense riddled, and plain stupid measures the so called professionals have attempted in coming up with non-injectable opioids. Am I missing something here? The truth of the matter is that it's still the same addictive opioid it was, and junkies will find a way to do them, regardless. The real problem is the fact that the opioid drugs are way too readily available. But no, the drug companies don't want us to stop the constant, heavy, distribution of their drugs, they just want to make them safer. Right...

If you're an innocent patient who suffered an unfortunate and painful ailment or injury of some kind, or a junkie as myself, what the hell is the difference if you're using them orally, injecting them, or snorting the shit? The bottom line is that you're hooked.

It almost reminds me of a television commercial that says "we're not the company that just makes an overabundance of opioids, we are the company that makes them safe." Very well, then...

What a crock of shit.

Another fact is that every penny that goes into all of the meetings, the research, and promotional lip service that's done by the drug companies, and the government commissions, are at the end of the day, passed on to us anyway. So why not create all of the smoke and mirrors trying to appear to be so concerned about the abuses. All the while, the drugs are going out the back door like a tsunami.

Just think, if instead of all of the money spent on meetings about warning labels, and other useless publications or warnings, would have been put into a dispenser, similarly to what I mentioned.

The bottom line seems to be that we've exhausted all other measures in stopping opioid abuse, so at the very least, the data which could be available to medical professionals in determining future care and options, by way of a controlled dispenser, is actually a viable option.

Again, would this dispenser be a lot more expensive than our current bottling methods? Definitely. Could it be broken into, or stolen? Sure. However, would the monitoring database show clear evidence of use vs abuse, or theft? Absolutely.

My question is; do the drug companies really want to fight opioid abuse if it means taking a tremendous hit in their distribution of the stuff. I highly doubt it. If the lip service and diversion tactics by way of changing the drug formulas appear to be working by keeping the drugs flowing, I highly doubt anything will change.

Again, what the hell is the difference if someone injects, snorts, or takes 20 OxyContin a day orally, it's still 20 too many.

Now, if we could just get heroin dealers to agree to incur the cost of their dispensers.

There will always be a price for achieving some safeguards in opioid use and abuse. The real question is, how truly important and genuine is our commitment in getting our arms around this epidemic?

Now, if someone does create one of these dispensers, I want 10% of the royalties.

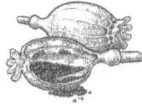

CHAPTER FORTY THREE

There are now cries for a commission to be set up by our government to address the current opioid epidemic before us. Do we really need more freakin commissions? Well, maybe in this case we do. And if they do in fact set one up, my suggestion would be my drug meter dispensers.

However, first and foremost, I would say that we fix the part of it, where a lot of it began.

First of all Purdue Pharma should have been shut down, with the guilty parties jailed. And, on that same line of inquisition into the whole mess, I say we follow the money.

What I am suggesting is that, in my opinion, on a hunch I have, is that there were possibly some payouts from Purdue Pharma to other people and/or agencies that assisted in this whole marketing scam that took place. I would say that there probably were people who were financially rewarded for favors in helping the drug company in their cause. Possibly in the way of suggesting that opioid addiction was overblown, and assisted in pushing the message out in a way to persuade physicians to escalate opioid prescribing. Namely OxyContin.

It's just too damn coincidental that the same year that Oxy-Contin was approved, just happened to be when the big push was set in place for physicians to treat pain more compassionately. Very interesting, and very telling, I'd say. Follow that money trail my friend.

Remember that I am a layperson with limited education, however, even I see why our healthcare system is such a dysfunctional mess, to the point of being detrimental to its patients. It is absolutely ridiculous seeing the circus that these clowns in these agencies are running.

What I see are a small number of physicians, who are seemingly wannabe politicians or executive businessmen, dictating what is good or bad medicine. They seem to be throwing in their 2cents (which results in, we the people, having to pull money out of our asses, that none of us have.) in the hopes of being big shots, and thrusting their will on the physicians who are trying to care for their patients, and for most of these wannabes, I am willing to bet, haven't touched a patient in years. Yet they dictate what is good, and bad medicine, with the end stage being the justification of their position. What a joke! And you wonder why our healthcare system is so horrendously dysfunctional, and costs through the roof?

When is someone in the position of authority going to wake the hell up, and pull the plug on this government style run circus, they call administrative excellence. To quote Vince Lombardi; "What the hell is going on out here!"

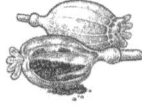

CHAPTER FORTY FOUR

There are different schools of thought on how to sway doctors from supposedly making people dependent on opiates. First of all, is this actually happening? Absolutely. However, is this really common? Absolutely not.

With proper education in as far as patient awareness before, during, and after, opioid prescribed patients are in the care of a physician, I honestly believe the extended agony of dependency can be eliminated. With the understanding that if the same patient has the addictive gene, then you'll more than likely see it in their actions during and following the time of opioid usage. There are usually symptoms that mirror the malcontent patient, whereas the pain is still present, beyond the average healing period. It could also be true that it would still be a painful process of recovery from the said injury that would linger beyond the norm. Every individual reacts differently to pain and the healing process, but that is where non-opioid medication becomes the necessity.

Ibuprofen is one in particular that works very well. But, I guarantee that once the word "Ibuprofen" comes out of the mouth of a physician, to an "at risk" kind of person, as myself, I promise that the proverbial wall of defense will go up immediately. And then it goes from defensive, to an offensive approach, by stating that he or she already tried that, and the pain is still unbearable. Well, to quote my 96 year old mother, "tough toenails".

In all seriousness, there are many of the said type of patients that do honestly carry symptoms of pain, whether real, or imagined, it is there just the same. That is definitely something that still needs to be addressed, whether it through chiropractic care, psychotherapy, anti-depressants, or even anti-epileptic medications. If all else fails, maybe it's time to bite the bullet and send them to the Methadone clinic.

If we look at opioid abuse from a Birdseye view, and closely analyze the various characteristics of what an "at risk" personality could be, you would no doubt see a number of categories. However, I honestly believe you will find that the vast majority of opioid abusers are people that are just plain discontent with life itself.

Though no patient who may have been medically administered opioids for an extended period, such as six months or more, that would be immune to the possibility of opiate dependency. However, there are definitely those of us who would be defiant in relinquishing our right to continue our opioid medication.

Obviously, many factors come into play when medical professionals determine the length of time a patient is prescribed opiates. There are injuries that are extremely painful, especially during the healing process, and each person's progress of mending differs.

Opioids certainly have been, are now, and no doubt may always be, the most effective substance in treating pain, as sure as the sun rises in the east, and sets in the west.

If there are any benefits, albeit they could even be defined as benefits, which came about from my years of floundering throughout life as a full-fledged opioid abuser, is my determination in finding alternative measures to treat pain.

During my initial stages of recovery from opioid addiction, I battled various aches and pains, that I never knew existed. More than likely, many of them were probably just phantom pains, It's just that the previous ten plus years, I hadn't really remembered experiencing pain of any sort, including psychological pain. I was just that oblivious to all of reality.

Some of the alternative measures I began to experiment with were ones like, trigger point injections, which became a saving grace of sorts for me. I had originally been plagued with back problems, which reared their ugly head, when I was clear of painkillers. It seemed every ache and pain was magnified tenfold. Some of it real pain, and surely some phantom pains, which that monkey was still attempting to point out. That son of a bitch never did leave, and probably never will.

Nowadays, in my attempts to ease my pains that do come about, without entertaining the thought of opioids being an option, I use things such as, acupuncture, hot and cold compresses, lime juice, and even rubbing dirt on it, as my mother would suggest. I just knew that I somehow needed to find a way that would help eliminate pain without opiates, or other narcotics.

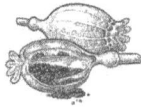

CHAPTER FORTY FIVE

In writing about the subject of opioids, and looking back, I realized it had become the most memorable and cherished relationship I ever encountered during my lifetime. It was like everything else I became enamored with in life, which for some reason, also seemed to be one of challenge, passion, and even treachery, this dysfunctional man I am. I just always seemed to want more of something I fell in love with. And in my never ending pursuit of the ultimate pleasure, I of course found it to be opioids, unfortunately.

I believe that if we take a very close look at the very root of the whole issue with opioids, you will see behind it all, the ultimate kingpin. It is THE ULTIMATE wolf in sheep clothing, Satan himself, "The Angel of Light, Yet, the Father of Lies". Who, or what else could bring such peace and tranquility to the ultimate destruction of the existence of so many on this earth.

In reality, the Opium Poppy (Papaver Somniferum) in every fiber of its makeup, through and through, is good and pure, down to the very seed from which it commenced. It is the fallibility of the "human condition" which exists in every human being walking this earth, that gives opium, one of the most useful and prominent discoveries ever introduced to the field of medicine, the aura of a horrible stain.

Unfortunately it's a very sad fact that some people, such as myself, who happen to possess a malfunctioning brain, flawed DNA, or just possibly an overbearing selfishness, are the very persons, who have created the stain that foreshadows the subject of opium.

The fact is that opiates are here to stay, and rightfully so. Again, there just isn't any treatment of pain and suffering that pale in comparison to opiates. The real problem that exists with opioids is when the "human condition" and free will come into the picture. And, it's the brain that gets the final say in making the choice of abusing opioids. It's a choice, and the determination of feel good vs the actual necessity in what opioids actual makeup offers. It's precisely like the old saying of "too much of a good thing gone badly"

As I look back at the history of my life it could very well be that I could have become the one and only person to actually come upon what mankind has been in endless pursuit of, the Fountain of Youth. But, sure enough, with my luck, I would end up drowning in the son of a bitch, and never live to tell anyone of my discovery. It's just the way my life always seemed to play out, with a never ending pursuit of selfish pleasures.

Throughout my travels, living on the dark and treacherous road of insanity during my lifetime, I somehow luckily survived, whereas so many before me, had not. For this, I am truly grateful, and I now find myself indebted to life itself, with a feeling of obligation to give back to society, what I stole from it, for so many years.

In closing, I need to say that there is that part of me that would like to say I am uniquely different from anyone else. I would like to inspire each and every one by telling you that I am one of the last, living, "Mighty Morphine Power Rangers" and that I endured the misery of addiction like no one else walking this earth. But the sobering fact is that I am no more unique, and not much different than anyone else in this thing we call recovery.

I am in fact just a very little piece of the puzzle in the road to recovery. But, it is this that which makes me so very much an important part in the scope of great hope that the 12 Step programs offer those who suffer from this disease.

I always want to remember, and may I never forget, the people before us that have paved the way for all of the fortunate people here today. It was through the sacrifice of way too many that have unfortunately suffered and even died, and those who have ultimately invested in our being here (somewhat) sane and sober today.